Textbook for
CHILDBIRTH EDUCATORS

SECOND EDITION

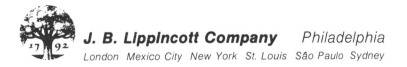

J. B. Lippincott Company   *Philadelphia*
London Mexico City New York St. Louis São Paulo Sydney

Sponsoring Editor: Paul Hill
Manuscript Editor: Rosanne Hallowell
Indexer: Julie Schwager
Art Director: Tracy Baldwin/Earl Gerhart
Designer: Ellen Sklar
Production Supervisor: J. Corey Gray
Compositor: Caledonia Composition
Printer/Binder: R. R. Donnelley & Sons Company

Cover photograph made possible through the generous cooperation of
Booth Maternity Center, Philadelphia, Pennsylvania

Second Edition

6 5 4 3 2 1

Library of Congress Cataloging in Publication Data

Hassid, Patricia.
  Textbook for childbirth educators.

  Bibliography: p.
  Includes index.
    1. Childbirth—Study and teaching.   2. Natural
childbirth—Study and teaching.   I. Title.
[DNLM: 1. Labor.   2. Natural childbirth.   3. Obstetrics—
Education.   WQ 18 H355t]
RG973.H37   1984   618.2′4   83-16239
ISBN 0-397-54469-3

PREFACE

Five years have passed since the first edition of *Textbook for Childbirth Educators* was published to furnish a standard reference work for childbirth instructors. During that time, changes have occurred and controversies have evolved within the maternal–child health field. No matter where we as childbirth educators may stand on a given issue, it is essential that we examine both sides in order to function as valid professional resource persons for the expectant parents with whom we interact. It is to help meet this need that I wrote the second edition.

One change discussed extensively in this edition is the rise in the rate of cesarean births. An entirely new chapter is devoted to cesarean birth classes, with a part of Chapter 7 devoted to inclusion of cesarean birth preparation in the regular childbirth preparation class.

New and different theories of pain perception have come and gone since the original work which was based on an understanding of gate control theory, but none have better served to explain the effectiveness of psychoprophylaxis. Thus, the psychoprophylaxis section has been left intact, with expansion to include new understandings of the role played by the endorphins.

Techniques have, for the most part, remained constant and effective. When confronted with variations of technique or new exercises that we may wish to add to our programs, it is important for us to evaluate for ourselves whether the new idea will be safe; sensible in terms of what we know about the physiology of pregnancy and labor; and at least as effective as the modality we are already using. Finally, we need to decide if the new technique or exercise will accomplish our objective. An example of this assessment process is in the discussion of the new "exhalation" pushing for the second stage of labor in Appendix A.

I wish that I could thank each of you individually who have taken the trouble to communicate to me all of your ideas for making this text more useful to you as you start out teaching, or as you attempt to improve your program. This book is not only *for* you, it is *of* you, and your contributions are gratefully acknowledged.

Patricia Hassid, R.N., B.A., M.Ed.

Preface to the First Edition

Knowledge of childbearing and parenting is increasing all the time. New technologies are being introduced into obstetric practice almost daily. Childbirth educators owe it to themselves and to their students to keep pace.

This book grew out of the need for a single text to be used in conjunction with programs for the preparation of childbirth educators. It incorporates teaching considerations with methodology. Many books on the market espouse one type of childbirth preparation or another, but none appear to have been written with the needs of the childbirth *educator* in mind.

An up-to-date reference on current obstetric practice, the book includes as well chapters on the neurophysiology of pain as it is presently understood and on preparation for variations of labor. There are special chapters on developing and implementing one's own childbirth preparation program and on presenting specific teaching techniques and strategy, as well as a suggested class outline for effective teaching. The basic orientation is psychoprophylaxis (PPM or Lamaze), but a review of other approaches to childbirth preparation is included.

This text is intended for use by both experienced and would-be educators. Those who are not nurses but wish to become professionals in this field should prepare themselves according to the requirements of their sponsoring agency. Nurses who want to enter the childbirth education field and physical therapists who have gained obstetric experience should prepare by attending organized teacher programs. Such programs help to crystallize one's thinking and to facilitate understanding of the underlying theory, and they offer opportunities to practice and perfect technique. The experience of learning in a group setting with opportunity for role playing, practice teaching, and feedback will enhance teaching potential.

Experienced educators should continue to expand their knowledge and to develop professionally by attending professional workshops and conferences and by taking continuing education courses. In addition to the new information acquired, interaction with other childbirth educators can be beneficial. Exposure to different approaches also helps to broaden perspectives. To keep abreast of current thinking and practice, one should belong to professional associations and read professional journals such as the Journal of Obstetrical, Gynecological and Neonatal Nursing (JOGN) and the American Journal of Maternal Child Nursing (MCN).

I am most grateful to my colleagues in the Council of Childbirth Education Specialists, Inc., Constance Castor and Polly DeSanto, who generously gave of their time and advice to bring this book to fruition.

Special thanks is also due to Susan E. Ralston for her ideas and suggestions and to the staff of Harper & Row, who patiently gave support in the many months it took to complete the book.

Lastly, I am deeply appreciative of the staunch support received from my wonder family, Debbie, Dan, and most especially my best friend and husband, who always urges me to be the best that I can be. He started me on the path to childbirth preparation when, as a young obstetrical resident, he came home excited at have witnessed a prepared couple actively participating in the birth of their child.

Patricia Hassid, R.N., B.A., M.Ed.

CONTENTS

Textbook for
CHILDBIRTH
EDUCATORS

Why is Childbirth Preparation Necessary?

Until fairly recent times, the concern of the health care professional involved with the childbearing experience has been limited to the physical safety of the mother and infant. Now that the mortality rate has dropped to an all-time low (although at least 15 countries have a lower mortality rate than the United States), attention has turned to making childbearing a psychologically rewarding experience as well as physically safe. Preparation for the stresses and strains of the perinatal period, as well as emotional support throughout, is one way of achieving this aim.

Birth should take its place among the other normal events in the psychologic, sexual, and social development of the woman. It needs to be integrated into her personal life cycle as well as the developmental cycle of her family if she and her husband are to grow from the experience and be ready for parenting. Childbearing is a time of stress and change for every family member as old relationships evolve into new and roles are reshaped.

This chapter examines some of the elements of the maturational crises of childbirth and their impact on all family members. We discuss how childbearing behavior is determined and how psychological care and support for the mother in the Western way of birth leave much to be desired. Finally, we take a look at family-centered maternity care and the emergence of the demand for change.

Childbirth: A Time of Crisis

First Pregnancy

Let us begin by clarifying the context in which we will be using the term *crisis*. Parad has given us this definition: "Maturational . . . crises are periods of marked physical, psychological, and social change that are characterized by common disturbances in thought and feeling."[4] At these critical periods, when the person is poised between growth and regression, integration and fragmentation, the opportunity arises for growth and development. However, ". . . the tasks inherent in the crisis itself must be faced and marked with a reasonable degree of effectiveness if the next maturational stage (in this case, parenting) is to yield its full potential for growth and development."[9]

For the couple bearing their first child, customary problem-solving mechanisms may be inadequate because of the couple's inexperience. Our task as care agents is to help them evoke new coping mechanisms that will serve to strengthen their adaptive capacity.

The First Trimester

Motivations for pregnancy vary widely. Couples may wish to prove their adult status or their freedom from childhood ties. They may be responding to cultural or familial expectations that everyone has, loves, or wants children. The husband may feel the need to prove his masculinity. The wife may want to prove her own capability and may picture herself as the "earth mother," serenely suckling her young. Sometimes, especially in the case of single women who choose to become pregnant, the woman may be approaching the age at which she feels delay would be irresponsible because of the increased risk of abnormality or complication.

Whatever the motivation for the pregnancy and however eagerly it is anticipated, the expectant parents feels a certain amount of ambivalence when the pregnancy is confirmed. Their concerns may center around timing or finances, or they may worry about their relationship and the changes that will occur in their lifestyle. They may share their concerns with each other, or feeling some vague sense of disloyalty to the coming baby or to the mate, they may keep their worry to themselves.

For the woman, her first baby is a final step away from childhood. Her "some time in the future" has become her "right now!"—shocking in its immediacy.[6] Her self-concept changes while she tests the reality of her situation. The girl/wife/playmate must become woman/wife/mother, a new and frightening idea. She knows herself as she is, but wonders who she may become. We commonly identify ourselves by our relationships with others and by how we structure our time, yet these foundations are the very ones that become shifting and unstable in the primigravida.[6]

The sense of discontinuity between the person one was and the person one will be is often reflected in moodiness and somatic complaints: nausea, morning sickness, extreme fatigue. The pregnancy cannot be seen or experienced in the early weeks except through these physical signs that serve to confirm its presence. The woman's task in this trimester is to work through her ambivalence toward being pregnant.

The Second Trimester

By the second trimester, the woman has usually begun to resolve some of these conflicts. The pregnancy has become obvious and therefore real. Fetal movements can be felt, confirming the presence of the child. The woman's mood becomes more introspective as, in her effort to adapt, she dreams of her child, its future looks and personality.

This fantasizing serves an important function in the expectant mother's psychological acceptance of her child. As professionals, we can help her to structure her fantasy by allowing her to listen to fetal heart tones, offering her books and baby names, using illustrated teaching aids, and generally being open to hearing about her daydreams. In this way, too, we may gain some knowledge of how she imagines herself as a mother.

One area for potential problems is that of increasing dependency. Women value their independence, especially now with the women's movement pointing out the multitude of ways in which women are assigned the role (in the words of Simone de Beauvoir) of the "second sex." Pregnancy, however, brings a sense of dependency that increases throughout the childbearing cycle, often causing the woman to become moody and fearful for her hard-won independence. She needs reassurance that this is a normal part of pregnancy and does not denote any lasting personality change.

By mobilizing her family to fulfill the woman's need to be nurtured, we are ensuring that she will have ample reserves to nurture in turn her forthcoming infant.[1,5]

The Third Trimester

By the third trimester, the pregnant woman's anxiety centers around thoughs about herself as a mother and about the newborn. Such thoughts as "Will I be a good mother?", "Will I be able to love my baby?", and "Will my baby be perfect? (Am I capable of producing a perfect baby?)" are typical. There is also a growing concern about how her mate will respond in his new role. She wonders if she can depend upon his being there when she needs him and if he will still love her in her new role.

Anxiety about her own ability to cope with the crisis of labor and birth on an adult level is always present to some extent but may be suppressed. These fears are very real and include fear of the unkown, of pain, and of disgracing herself, as well as doubts about her own ability to parent.

These worries reach a crescendo in the third trimester and, coupled with a heightened sense of dependency, lead to insecurity, mood swings, and lowered self-esteem.

The expectant father, meanwhile, may be experiencing his own doubts about his ability to provide for his increasing family. This is especially true if parenthood will mean the loss of his wife's income. He may wonder how he will continue to respond to the moody creature that his wife has become and if he will ever again see the woman he married. His wife's expanding body may have necessitated a change in their usual sex practices, and he may wonder if their sex life will ever again be the same. Although the coming infant has less reality for the expectant father, he too may wonder about his ability to be a good parent and if he will love his child. Not realizing that he needs to mourn the loss of the carefree preparental state in order to accept and make ready for his parenting role, he may fear that any resentment of his unborn infant is unnatural. Unless he comes into a group with other expectant or experienced fathers, he has little access to sharing these concerns.

When expecting their first grandchild, the expectant grandparents, to a lesser degree, are also undergoing a change in their self-image. Not only are their children about to give tangible evidence of adult status, but they see themselves in a new light. Most of us conceptualize grandparents as being like our own grandparents, which in this youth oriented culture translates *Old*. Each expectant grandparent must reevaluate his relationship with grown children, who suddenly have become grown adults.

Subsequent Pregnancies

We have concentrated primarily upon changes that occur with the first pregnancy. The same needs and anxieties are present in subsequent pregnancies, although usually less accentuated. The expectant mother has the same need for nurturing as she did the first time, but unfortunately these needs are less likely to be met because those around her feel that she has, after all, been through it all before.

Subsequent pregnancies have an effect upon all family relationships. The time of stress continues and increases throughout pregnancy, childbirth and the neonatal period while new roles and relationships are being defined. Siblings may resent the newborn, and parents may find themselves torn between their natural sympathetic understanding of the older child and their strong desire to protect the newborn. Crisis intervention in the form of counseling or well-thought-out prenatal preparation can influence this opportunity for growth in a mentally healthy direction.

Culturally Conditioned Behavior

Primitive Behavior

Human birthing behavior can never be natural in the sense of being innate, for although the fetus must follow its preordained pathway into the outside world, the behavior of the parents is culturally determined. Even in the animal world, the animal cannot be said to "know" how to behave prior to giving birth. Rather the animal mother exhibits some innate reactions to physiologic and adaptive needs as demonstrated by the licking behavior of animals high on the mammalian scale.

The parturient cat, for example, begins to lick herself prior to giving birth, altering usual washing patterns by emphasizing the nipple line and pelvic regions. Studies have shown that pregnancy causes increased sensitivity in these areas. During birth her washing of the genital area includes ingestion of some of the birth fluids, which stimulates her licking behavior further. If some of these fluids spill onto the birth surface, she also licks this area. As the kittens emerge covered with amniotic fluid, her tongue stimulates them to breathe as she continues to lick them. In addition, the licking of her offspring binds the mother to them. If she has licked them, she will retrieve them and gather them in close to her nipples.[8] Eventually she eats the placenta and cord.

Safety and privacy are needed for giving birth in both the animal world and in our own. Many animals build nests; other simply withdraw until the birth has taken place. Some, such as the elephant or dolphin, surround themselves with other females of their species who protect the mother while she is vulnerable, driving off intruders and supporting the newborn until the mother can take over this function.

As young humans mature, they are conditioned by their culture to expect certain types of adult behavior in certain situations, such as pregnancy and birth. Such behavior is far from being instinctive in that it is always subject to modification according to what is necessary for the survival of the neonate and the value system of the culture.

In isolated cultures, the customs and mores surrounding birth give the expectant couple ritualized roles to play. While these rituals may not have any actual effect upon the process of birth, they do provide culture support. The parents know exactly what is expected of them and how they should behave. For example, the practice of considering the new mother "unclean" or taboo until a ritual purification has taken place (usually 4-5 weeks after parturition) may seem nonsensical to us, but it does give the new mother privacy, time to become sensitized to the needs of her newborn, and time to recuperate. It also grants her freedom from everyday tasks such as cooking, tending the household, and so forth. She receives nurturing from others who must take over these tasks for as long as she is unclean. Gradually the restrictions are lifted, and the new mother is eased into her new role.[5]

Although in some primitive societies the husband is expected to perform the **couvade** and so draw the attention of evil spirits away from his wife, in most societies childbearing is the responsibility of the woman or of the extended family. In many societies she is tended by other women who have borne children. In others, she withdraws by herself to give birth; for example, Eskimo women withdraw to the water's edge to give birth because it is the one place where they are not surrounded by others.

Behavior in Western Society

Cultural and familial support is far less evident in Western society. Frequently the young couple live far from their own families and must look for support only to each other or to their busy obstetrician, who is chiefly concerned with the physical health of mother and child. In addition, childbearing has assumed an aura of mystery, far removed from the normal cycle of life, so that the couple have no example of normal childbearing behavior to use as a pattern. The removal of the childbearing experience from the couple's marriage cycle, which began with the removal of the birth to the hospital, was completed when the woman herself was removed from awareness by the administration of general anesthesia.

The responsibility for the birth, which was gladly given up by the 19th century woman who wanted only to be freed from pain, was relegated to the physician or to the institution in which the woman delivered. There was a shift in emphasis from the woman's giving birth to the physician's delivering an infant under sterile conditions. Having been given the responsibility and thereby the control of the birth, the medical community assumed an increasingly parental stance. The mother became more passive and felt unable or incompetent to effect the birth process, which enhanced her feelng of helplessness. The question of power and to whom the birth belongs (woman? family? physician? hospital?) is controversial and is one of the factors that has led to the recent demand for change.

Emergence of the Demand for Change

The demand for change can be seen in all areas: social, political, sexual, economic. In part this is due to increased education and public awareness. Tribal societies do not change because they are not exposed to new ideas, but there has been unprecedented change in our own society since radio and television have become widely available. The rise of consumerism has meant that people demand an increasingly active role in all the important events of their lives, including the childbearing experience.

Hospital Care

In the past, hospitals were largely unresponsive to change. The almost universal use of large amounts of analgesics and sedatives for labor made it mandatory for the parturient to receive custodial care while she labored, if only to prevent injury. In common with the admission procedures of other institutions that offer custodial care, the hospital admission procedure included removal of clothing and personal belongings, separation from family, and the replacement of a name with a number. The demoralizing effect of these procedures is frequently cited by activists in their demand for a more humanized birth experience.

Happily, hospitals are today reevaluating policies in response to consumer demands, as well as changing standards of obstetric practice in relation to medication and anesthesia. Two decades ago medical attention was focused primarily on the comfort of the mother, whereas today, because we are more aware of the long-range effects of maternal medications on the infant, attention has shifted to the welfare of the infant. Concomitantly there has been a growing awareness of the emotional aspects of the childbirth experience and their impact on parental attachment in the perinatal period.

Family-Centered Care

Family-centered maternity care, of which childbirth education is a part, has been an outgrowth of our awareness of the need for change. In this type of care, the family is regarded as an integral unit. Every effort is made to increase the involvement of family members and thereby strengthen mutual support.

Research on maternal attachment and maternal deprivation is being done by such writers as Kennel and Klaus who are specifically investigating the effects of early separation of mother and child.[3] Brazelton writes on "What Childbirth Drugs Can Do to Your Child" in a magazine for the lay public.[2] These writers find that there is a critical time for bonding to take place between the mother and her infant during the first postpartal hour. If they are separated from each other during this sensitive period, the attachment process will be delayed and perhaps subtly affected for a long time to come.

The bonding of the infant to its parents may also be affected when the child is suffering the aftereffects of medication given to the mother during labor. Since the infant's immature system cannot metabolize and excrete the medication for a period of several days to several weeks, his responses to fondling as well as to nursing may be sluggish.[2] Because the parent–infant bonding process is dependent upon reciprocal responses, by the time the infant is alert and ready to be fully responsive to his parents overtures, the optimal time may have passed.

These harbingers of the changes to come are all pediatricians and child psychologists rather than obstetricians. Unfortunately, as we concentrate on pregnancy, childbirth, or the newborn, we still have too little concern for the emerging family as a whole.

Childbirth Education

Childbirth education helps the couple work through the "problem" of labor cooperatively in a manner that will be satisfying to both of them: it gives them coping skills and encourages mutual participation. In childbirth classes, feelings about the labor and the coming baby are discussed in an atmosphere of total acceptance. If negative feelings can be expressed, they have a better chance of being resolved. Techniques for coping with the rigors of labor are given, and the couple is urged to practice intensively the techniques they later will apply to the particular type of labor that occurs.

Solving the "problem" of labor increases the couple's problem-solving ability in the postpartum period, as their success gives them confidence. Helping a couple toward an active, independent role in the childbearing experience by emphasizing their ability to resolve difficulties and stressing flexibility enhances their potential for working together in many other ways.

The couple's cooperation with every member of the childbirth team is strongly advocated to mobilize support for their efforts.[7] This crisis intervention involves not only the childbirth educator (who will only see the couple for a very limited time) but also the clinic or office nurse, the labor and delivery room nurse, and, of course, the physician or midwife. To be effective, the supportive milieu must prevail throughout.

The attitudes of each member of the childbirth team can influence the psychological outcome of the birth experience. If negative feelings about the experience, their own behavior, or the reactions of others are left to be resolved by the new parents, it delays their ability to give their full attention to the next task in their developmental cycle, that of parenting. They need to be reassured that they have "done well." It is important to remember that "doing well" should mean that their efforts were not meaningless. The use or nonuse of medically indicated intervention is not a criterion for success, and the new parents may have to be reminded of this.

This strong psychological support is continued after delivery by the postpartum and nursery nurses. Positive feedback about the new parents' ability to care for the infant as well as explanations and demonstrations of infant care are essential here. The new mother must be encouraged to be active in caring for herself and her newborn. Close observation of the interactions between parents and their newborn can often detect incipient problems.

Family-centered maternity care that includes rooming in enables the parents to become acquainted with their infant while still under the aegis of the hospital. Whereas during the final months of pregnancy their primary interest was in the labor and birth, now they are ready and anxious to know and learn everything they can about how to be parents.

Objectives of Preparation Programs

One of the optimal ways to implement a program of family-centered care is to begin with a well-thought-out childbirth preparation program. There are five overall objectives of childbirth preparation programs:

1. To provide a supportive milieu
2. To reduce anxiety
3. To provide factual information
4. To provide practical tools for labor
5. To keep the focus on current concerns

Table 1-1 provides a sample class outline incorporating these objectives.

Providing a Supportive Milieu

Providing a supportive milieu is one of the most important functions of childbirth preparation programs. This can be done by encouraging communication between the couple and all members of the childbirth team

Table 1-1. **Sample Class Outline in Psychoprophylaxis**

Class	Content	Rationale
I	Introduce self, give background.	Sets tone, welcoming atmosphere
	Have students introduce themselves and state reasons for coming to class.	Gives idea of attitudes and knowledge; establishes mutuality of concern
	Discuss course content and goals.	Develops awareness of goals of instructor and student tasks
	Give overview of course content.	Establishes contact, correct expectation
	Present basic concepts of psychoprophylaxis and how it affects pain and the childbirth experience.	Promotes understanding, essential for informed active participation
	Discuss menstrual cycle, process of conception, fetal development, physicial and emotional changes during pregnancy.	Increases awareness of normalcy of pregnant state, reinforces reality of baby
	Give overview of labor and delivery.	Helps to structure realistic expectation
	Teach physical fitness exercises.*	Improves posture, muscle tone, circulation, comfort
	Teach controlled relaxation preparatory exercise.	Develops awareness of tension and relaxation; develops idea of team effort for labor; provides foundation for later techniques
II	Review and ask for questions relating to materials presented in Class I.	Reinforces concepts presented in Class I
	Review physical fitness exercises.	Reinforces ability
	Review controlled relaxation preparatory exercise.	Reinforces ability; emphasizes strengths and teamwork
	Add practice drill.	Provides opportunity to practice ability to release tension under stress; adds new skills to those previously learned
	Discuss early labor, onset, and early active labor; include mood, contractions, sensations, coaching role.	Develops knowledge begun in previous overview of labor
	Introduce two basic respiratory techniques.	Easy-to-learn basic steps for ready learner acceptance
III	Review and ask for feedback on materials presented previously.	Reinforces knowledge through repetition; corrects misunderstandings
	Review rationale and observe skills in performing controlled relaxation, and preparatory and practice exercises.	Reinforces ability
	Add controlled relaxation in the lateral position.	Builds on previously learned skills
	Review rationale and observe skills of two basic respiratory techniques.	Reinforces ability
	Add respiratory progression for labor.	Builds on previously learned skill
	Concurrently, discuss active labor and transition phase.	Teaches how techniques apply to labor

(continued)

Table 1-1. **Sample Class Outline in Psychoprophylaxis** *(continued)*

Class	Content	Rationale
	Explain possible variations of first stage: (1) back labor, (2) medications, (3) fetal monitor (if applicable), (4) induction or implementation.	Develops awareness of possible variations to reduce anxiety
IV	Review material presented in Class III and ask for questions; include entire first stage of labor and coaching role.	Reinforces knowledge through repetition; corrects misunderstandings
	Review and observe respiratory progression.	Reinforces skills; makes it possible to identify problems
	Present second stage of labor; include physical and emotional factors, work, mood, contractions; emphasize coaching role.	Reinforces knowledge from overview; adds new knowledge; excites expectant parents about their own role in birth of their child
	Teach expulsion technique.	Provides understanding of mechanism of second stage and how correct positioning will aid in the expulsion
	Review controlled relaxation, especially in lateral position for back labor.	Ends the class with previously learned and integrated material
V	Review entire labor including hospital admission, delivery room procedures, coaching role and all techniques (possibly using role playing).	Reinforces learning; helps to identify problems
	Discuss 3rd stage of labor, variations of 2nd & 3rd stages.	Creates realistic expectation
	Present and discuss cesarean birth using visual aides.	Adds to previous knowledge Anticipatory guidance for unexpected outcome
VI	Review all techniques and labor as necessary.	Provides an opportunity for last-minute questions
	Discuss in depth the postpartum period: physical recovery, psychological adjustments, needs and feelings of mother and father.	Prepares students for postpartum stress, helping to establish coping mechanisms
	Discuss appearance and needs of newborn.	Prepares new parents for immaturity of newborn
	Teach postpartum exercises, physical fitness.	Emphasizes the continuing need for physical fitness

*Detailed instructions for teaching the exercises may be found in Appendix A.

and by stressing cooperation as well as the individual importance of each team member.

The childbirth educator must act as a **facilitator** to ensure that the team functions smoothly. She must know how the labor and delivery units function at the particular hospitals where her students will deliver, and she should let the units know of any potential problems. She should be familiar with the routines of the physicians who will deliver her students, but this may be impossible if the class is large and made up of patients from many different physicians. However, communication between physician and patient is increased if the patient herself asks her physician about particular routines. The importance of communication between physician and patient seems obvious, but there is often surprisingly little communication, either because the woman is timid about asking, she forgets, or the physician is rushed. Giving her specific questions to ask may help her to overcome this problem.

Some childbirth classes require written consent from the physician before the expectant mother can be accepted into class. Although a permission slip has no legal value, it has the advantage of opening the topic of childbirth preparation for discussion with the physician. Sometimes the mother is asked to have her physician provide a note; other instructors furnish a written form for the physician to sign. A form such as the one in Figure 1-1 also alerts the physician to the fact that the instructor needs to know if the woman must restrict activity, in which case the instructor might limit herself to teaching this particular woman. relaxation and respiratory techniques only.

To ensure the smooth functioning of the childbirth team, each member of the team must have a clear idea of what his or her role will be, as well as an understanding of the roles that will be fulfilled by other team members.

The expectant mother is responsible for following her physician's instructions on her prenatal care, for coming to class, for asking questions that are of concern to her, and for learning the various techniques for labor

JANE DOE, R. N.
PREPARATION FOR CHILDBIRTH

Address
Phone #

Ms. _____ has my permission to attend class, and to participate in prenatal exercises.

Restrictions as noted □

No Restrictions □

Signed: _____ M.D.

FIG. 1-1. Sample professional card and permission slip.

and practicing them diligently. She is responsible for her own behavior and application of the techniques during labor.

The labor coach is responsible for attending class with the expectant mother, for asking questions about issues that are of concern to him, and for using the discipline of repetitive practice with the expectant mother to begin the conditioning process. He should see his role as one of helping her to use the techniques that she has learned. In labor his role is that of supporter and comforter. Using the verbal cues that they have practiced together, he reinforces the learned responses. He encourages her and works with her to achieve a satisfying birth experience.

The physician or midwife is responsible for directing the woman's care and making all medical decisions. In the prenatal period the physician discusses labor with the expectant mother or couple so that there is agreement on management of the labor as long as it is normal. Ideally, the physician is supportive of the couple's desire to share the birth experience and reinforces their efforts in the labor period.

The labor room nurse is the liason between the hospital and the couple. She explains procedures and offers encouragement and assistance when necessary. She is also responsible for monitoring the mother and baby. Ideally, she familiarizes herself with what the couple are trying to accomplish and is able to take over the coaching role for short periods to give the coach a break.

The childbirth educator can offer an orientation program to the hospital staff if her program is new to the area. One approach might be to ask the obstetrical supervisor how she feels students can best be prepared to function in the obstetric unit. This involves the supervisor and gives the educator some feedback on possible problem areas. Literature about the program or about the team approach to childbirth, such as reprints of "The Childbirth Team During Labor" could be distributed.[7]

Reducing Anxiety

Another goal of childbirth preparation programs is to reduce anxiety by giving the couple an opportunity to discuss their concerns in an atmosphere of acceptance. Understanding that other couples share their concerns will help to reduce the feeling of isolation and strengthen lateral supports. Acceptance of the variety of feelings and fears by the leader shows respect for each individual.

Providing Factual Information

A basic understanding of what is going on within the woman's body during pregnancy, labor, and the **postpartum** period provides a feeling of preparedness and calm. The more realistically the couple is able to structure their fantasy about labor and delivery, the better they will be prepared for its stresses.

Providing Practical Tools

Besides their physiological and psychological benefits (increased circulation and respiratory exchange, reduced fatigue, reduced perception of contractions as painful, confidence in ability to cope), the techniques are practical tools for coping with the discomforts of labor and delivery. They give couples a way to respond to the contractions by providing a model for behavior. Focusing the attention on performance of technique activates the woman's cognitive level of response. She must organize her behavioral responses.

Keeping the Focus on Current Concerns

People learn best what they desire to learn. If the educator is aware of the needs of expectant parents in the various partal periods, she can focus class content upon what is important at the moment. For example, women in the third trimester are less interested in infant care than they were in the second trimester. Being close to term, their overriding concern is how they will handle the labor and delivery.

These five generalized objectives provide a framework upon which course content can be assessed. The expectant woman or couple does not need to know everything the instructor knows. Knowledge of obstetric curiosities does not help the expectant couple, unless there is a possibility that they can cause or avoid them. The facts they need are those upon which they must make decisions or those that provide knowledge of or realistic expectations about the childbearing experience.

References

1. Benedek T: The psychosomatic implications of the primary unit: Mother–child. Child Family 8: 213, 1969
2. Brazelton TB: What childbirth drugs can do to your child. Redbook Magazine, Feb 1971
3. Klaus M, Kennell J: Maternal–Infant Bonding. St. Louis, CV Mosby 1976
4. Parad JH: Crisis Intervention: Selected Readings, p 73. New York, Family Service Association of America, 1965
5. Raphael D: The Tender Gift: Breastfeeding. Englewood Cliffs, NJ, Prentice Hall, 1973
6. Rubin R: Cognitive style in pregnancy. Am J Nurs 70:502–508, 1970
7. Sasmor J, Castor C, Hassid P: The childbirth team during labor. Am J Nurs 73:444–447, 1970
8. Schneirla TC, Rosenblatt JS, Tobach E: Maternal behavior in cats. In Rheingold HL (ed): Maternal Behavior in Animals. New York, John Wiley and Sons, 1963
9. Yoshioka R: Maturation crisis of childbearing. In Clark A: Maturational Crisis of Pregnancy, p 15. Honolulu, University of Hawaii, 1971

2

Pain and its Perception

Any book about childbirth must include a discussion of pain. Through the years, the search for a way to reduce childbirth pain has been secondary only to concern for the physical safety of mother and infant. One of the original goals of psychoprophylactic preparation was childbirth without pain.[2]

In the past there have been many theories concerning the neurophysiology of pain. These include such theories as specificity, which states that specific nerves carry only pain impulses and that there is a pain center in the brain whose function is to interpret pain.

Today we believe that the nerves that carry pain impulses also carry touch and pressure signals from the stimulated area to the spinal cord. A signal is relayed from these incoming nerves to the spinal cord fibers, which carry it up to the **thalamus**. There the signal is relayed to the cerebral cortex, where it is interpreted, and a response is made. The signal may be modified at any of these relays (Fig. 2-1).

The transmission of impulses may be interpreted as painful involves not only nerve fibers, cord, thalamus, and cerebral cortex, but also the systems involved in **affective** (emotional) and sensory activities, that is, the entire brain.[5] Although the various responses to the pain stimulus, as well as the variables that affect its interpretation and perception, can be discussed separately, it is essential to remember that pain is a unified process.

One of the most difficult tasks is to find an adequate definition of pain itself. The dictionary defines pain as a feeling of hurt. Everyone understands this definition, but each of us understands it differently. As a personal experience, pain can never be adequately communicated to others. We therefore interpret the words *hurt* or *pain* according to our own past experience with it.

Similarly, we are unable to judge pain in others except in terms of response. The identical stimulus may elicit a feeling of pain and a pain response in one person, yet cause little reaction in another. The difference lies in the individual's perception and interpretation of the stimulus.

A stimulus is defined as something that incites action, that is, any change in physical energy sufficient to be responded to by an organism. A

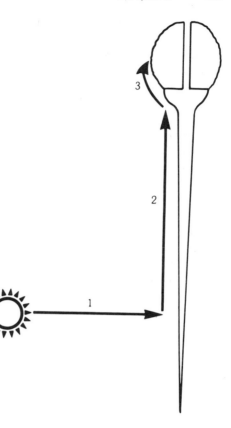

FIG. 2-1. Transmission system (1) Impulses travel from the site of **innervation** over sensory nerve fibers to the spinal cord. (2) Impulses travel up the cord to the thalamus and reticular formation. (3) Most impulses are relayed from the thalamus to the cerebral cortex for interpretation. Others are re-layed back down the cord to after incoming signals.

pain stimulus is generally considered to be one that produces or threatens to produce tissue damage, although this is not always the case (as in childbirth).

Neurologic Responses

The theory of neurologic response that is currently the most accepted is the gate control theory. Introduced in 1965 by Melzack and Wall it is broken down into four systems: transmission, gate control, central control, and action systems.[6]

Transmission System

The reaction to the stimulus is transmitted over sensory nerve fibers to the dorsal root ganglia, which enter the spinal cord. There the impulse is transmitted across the synapse and ascends by way of the lateral spino-thalamic tract to the thalamus.

There are numerous exceptions to this direct pathway, however. The innervation of the cord overlaps as the dorsal root ganglia enter the cord at various levels. In addition, although the lateral spinothalamic tract is the chief pathway for pain impulses, the impulse may ascend on more than one spinal tract.

Above the level of the cervical cord these sensory nerve pathways funnel together, and the majority end in the ventrolateral nucleus of the thalamus. Other branching collaterals go to the reticulated fibers in the brain stem, which then project the impulse back down the cord to alter response thresholds for incoming stimuli. From the thalamus, the pathways relay to the sensory cortex, which interprets stimuli and institutes appropriate responses. Continuous interaction takes place between the cortex, the thalamus, and reticular formation in the brain stem to organize and generate responses to pain signals and to initiate protective mechanisms.

Gate Control System

Impulses from the causal stimuli travel over sensory nerves from the viscera or periphery to the spinal cord. Within these nerves, the impulses may be carried either by the large-diameter fibers, which are relatively inactive in the absence of stimuli, or by the small-diameter fibers, which monitor the ongoing impulses related to **homeostasis**. The impulses carried by the large-diameter fibers rapidly activated the central transmission cells in the dorsal horn that carry the impulse up the cord; however, a blocking mechanism that inhibits the transmission of later impulses is quickly produced by chemical alteration of the **substantia gelatinosa**.

In contrast, the impulses carried by the small-diameter nerve fibers are initially slow to cause a reaction in the transmission cells. Unlike the impulses carried by the larger-diameter fibers, the effectiveness of these incoming signals is *enhanced* as they continue.

This modulating action takes place in the densely packed cells of the substantia gelatinosa, which surround the terminals of the incoming sensory nerve fibers and act upon their membrane potentials, thereby controlling the synaptic ability of the impulse before it can affect the transmission cells. Thus, we can see that although impulses from large-diameter fibers begin by being immediately effective, the feedback from reticulated fibers in the brain stem to the substantia gelatinosa causes the gating mechanism to hold a relatively closed position. If the impulses continue, adaptation begins to take place and the proportion of large-diameter fibers that are involved begins to diminish.

As the responses in the large-diameter fibers diminish and the proportion of small-diameter fiber impulses increases, the gate is forced into a more receptive position. The effectiveness of the impulse on the transmission cells is related directly to the ratio of small- and large-fiber activity (Fig. 2–2).

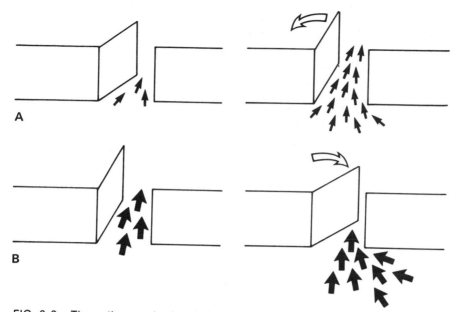

FIG. 2-2. The gating mechanism is influenced by the ratio of large to small fibers activated. (*A*) Impulses carried on small-diameter nerve fibers are initially ineffective in activating the gating mechanism. As impulses continue, their action is enhanced and the gate is held in a relatively *open* position. (*B*) Impulses traveling on large-diameter fibers are immediately effective, but feedback to substantia gelatinosa causes the gate to hold a relatively *closed* position.

Melzack and Wall propose that the three most significant features for pain are

1. The ongoing activity that precedes the stimulus (are large and small fibers already active?)
2. The stimulus-evoked activity (the number of fibers activated)
3. The balance of large *versus* small fibers activated

Central Control System

It has long been established that such central nervous system activities as anxiety, memory of previous experiences with pain, and directed attention give rise to descending (efferent) nerve impulses, which are capable of enhancing or inhibiting the flow of sensory stimuli. The central control trigger mechanism of the gate control system influences the terminals of afferent fibers at the earliest presynaptic level (*i.e.*, before synapse from sensory nerves to central transmission cells of the dorsal horn) before the action system is activated.

This mechanism may be triggered by ascending patterns in the dorsal column system, which have a rapid rate of rise within the spinal cord. This rapid rise time allows for the signal to be identified, evaluated, localized, and inhibited before slower rising signals have a chance to affect the action system. Thus, before a response is initiated, the incoming signals have already been modulated by the negative feedback from the central transmission cells and the central control trigger mechanism.

Action System

Once the output of the central transmission cells reaches a critical level, it triggers the action system, which is involved with the perception of and responses to pain. The person reacts in the more or less predictable fashion that is referred to as overt pain response (startle, withdrawal, inspection, crying out, *etc.*). Perceptual awareness changes as the person interprets the incoming sensation according to past experience, environment, and coping style. The interactions that evolve between the gate control and the action systems may take place at any level of the central nervous system, being set and reset as the incoming information is analyzed and acted upon by the brain.

The Endorphins

Ten years after Melzack and Wall first proposed the gate control theory, new horizons were opened by biochemical research into internally produced substances that have opiate-like effects on cerebral and neural functioning. Produced by neurosecretory cells, these hormones are generically known as endorphins, and act to influence the transfer of sodium ions through cell membranes. These substances are found throughout the body, but particularly in areas that mediate the neural transmission of pain. This regulatory effect appears to fit neatly into the central control system proposed by Melzack and Wall. With less than a decade of research behind us, our knowledge about the endorphins is scanty, but current research has opened up some exciting possibilities related to pain.

The endorphins affect both behavioral and physiological functions, such as respiration, blood pressure, appetite, bowel functioning, state of mind, and affect. That all the mammalian creatures studied were found to have receptors of endorphins in their central nervous system cells would seem to indicate a fundamental biological role. A number of researchers have found that the endorphins (like the opiates) provoke prolactin secretion, which is associated with feelings of pleasure, nurturing behavior, stimulation of lactation, and the suppression of the naturally occuring depressive substance, dopamine. The ability to induce these feelings of warmth, satisfaction, and the reduction of pain sensitivity suggests that the endorphins reward and reinforce behaviors that increase endorphin production, and explains the well-known tendency of the opiates to create dependency and habit-forming behavior (Fig. 2–3).[2]

One study reported significantly higher endorphin levels in laboring

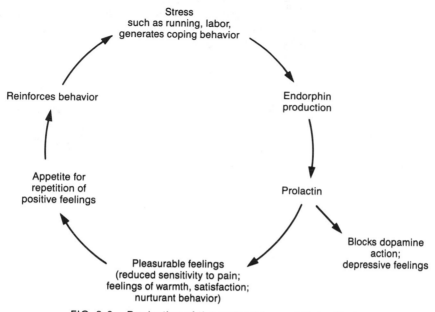

FIG. 2-3. Production of the endorphins and their effects.

and parturient women and in term infants who had just undergone the stress of labor, as well as in distance runners and joggers just after the stress of running. Conclusions were drawn relating the biologically important behaviors of production and nurturing of infants and the behavior of running to further suggest a natural reward system for those activities that evoke the production of endorphins.[2,3]

Demonstration of a possible use of endorphins for obstetric analgesia was perfomed in Japan, where beta-endorphin was injected by means of lumbar puncture to women in labor.[7] Results showed long-lasting effects in reduction of pain perception with no demonstrable change in fetal heart rate or Apgar scores. However, some side-effects were noted, including the presence of spinal headache in 10 out of the 14 women studied, and nausea and vomiting in 4 of the 14. This demonstration was important because of the association of analgesic effects in labor with increased endorphin levels. However, further studies are necessary before any conclusions can be drawn.

The relationship between endorphin levels, pain sensitivity, and nurturing behavior is complex, and reports in the literature are difficult to relate directly to the practice of the childbirth educator. Studies are either extremely limited in scope or are done on other than human species. We all know that our students demonstrate marked differences in sensitivity to pain in labor. It seems likely that individual variation in endorphin production is a major element in their overall tolerance and coping patterns. At this time we are unable to pinpoint precise behaviors that evoke endorphin production naturally other than active participation and coping behavior in such stressful activities as running and parturition.

Physiologic Responses

The physiologic changes that occur in response to pain stimuli are primarily related to the organism's preparation for action. These reactions are identical to those brought about by fear or anger and represent markedly heightened activity of the autonomic nervous system. Logically enough, the presence of fear or anger in addition to pain increases the intensity of the response.

The initial changes that take place include increases in pulse rate, circulating blood sugar, and blood flow to the larger striated muscles, as well as a decrease in blood flow to the viscera. Decreased gastric activity and secretion may lead to discomfort and vomiting. Increased alveolar ventilation causes increased oxygen consumption and can lead to hyperventilation. The increased blood flow to local striated musculature may lead to increased muscular tension.

Behavioral Responses

In discussing gross motor responses we must consider many variables that cannot be measured scientifically, for example, cognitive functioning, body image, and various personality characteristics.

It has been virtually impossible to separate pure pain responses from anxiety reactions. Partly because the mechanism of pain reaction prepares the person to withdraw from the noxious stimulus, failure to do so results in increased feelings of anxiety. Thus, a person's style of coping with anxiety directly relates to her ability to cope with pain.

Overt Responses

Overt behavioral responses to painful stimuli include withdrawal, increased tension, writhing, and verbalization. These are all responses that characterize a person in pain. We tend to judge the amount of pain being experienced by these overt reactions, sometimes forgetting that people differ widely in their interpretation of and responses to identical stimuli. It is desirable to distinguish between **pain threshold** and **pain tolerance,** because the relationship between these terms is frequently misunderstood. A person may say she has a "low pain threshold," meaning that her tolerance for pain is low. The threshold itself refers to the point at which the stimulus elicits a neurologic response. The tolerance level is the point at which the person no longer accepts the stimulus without making an active attempt at escape or verbalization. New studies have linked

individual differences in pain sensitivity to related differences in endorphin production levels.

In addition to expressing the person's need to escape painful stimuli,
overt pain reactions serve to communicate distress and rally support. Pain
response styles may reveal hidden needs, such as the need to be dependent or
to gain control over others. The name of this psychological game could be
expressed as "Look how much I suffer," or "See how brave I am."

It is important to remember that patterns of response to pain are a
result of childhood experiences. Small children cry out when they
experience pain, and if their parents come and "make it better," they are
reassured and feel safe. The reassurance and presence of a caring person are
the necessary components. Older children, however, might be told not to
make such a fuss. In this way feelings of ambivalence arise, and dependency
needs are mixed with guilt for seeking sympathy. Also, spanking children
when they are naughty reinforces the notion that pain is punishment for
wrongdoing.

The adult in pain experiences the same desire for some caring person
to come and "make it better." As pain increases, so does dependency and
regression, as may be readily surmised by the language of the person in
pain. For example, the laboring woman in the traditional labor room
situation typically begins by begging for relief from those around her. This
is followed by pleas to "Mamma" and to "God." If relief is not
forthcoming, she begins to blame herself (like the small child who
associates pain with punishment). Her promises to "be good" or to give up
something to escape the punishment of pain are heartrending. Finally, if it
seems that nothing is going to help, she withdraws into herself, sobbing
hopelessly.

The pain sensation, then, causes both escape and anxiety responses.
These responses become so associated that later evocation of one may also
elicit the other. In this way an affective response associated with pain may
cause a physiological one, or a behavioral response may serve as a stimuli
for other responses. This relationship is important to our comprehension
of how labor contractions may give rise to all of these pain responses,
although the stimulus does not produce or threaten to produce tissue
damage.

Anxiety and Coping Style

Emotional reactions to the experience of pain are also dependent upon
past conditioning. This includes such variables as the meaning that pain
has for the person and any anxiety about its cause and results. Anxiety
about possible injury, loss, or inability to cope with pain decreases the
ability to maintain control over behavior, and loss of control enhances
terror and the individual's self-image as a person in pain. It can be said,
therefore, that anxiety increases pain response and, conversely, that pain

response increases anxiety, especially if the behavior exhibited is unacceptable to the person's self-concept.

Cultural Variables

Familial and cultural background have a marked influence upon the behavior exhibited by the person in pain. Expressions of pain have various meanings, purposes, and levels of acceptance in different cultures.[6] For example, those with a Yankee background are far more inhibited in their overt expressions of pain than those of Italian or Semitic background. To the Yankee, pain is something to be endured in private. Gross displays of body language and emotion may be regarded as unseemly and unhelpful, and self-control may be viewed as the ideal. When pain is reported, it is likely to be mentioned simply as a useful symptom for diagnosis, without emotion. The Semitic and Italian groups, on the other hand, are more likely to employ public expression of their pain, this being culturally approved behavior designed to rally sympathy and assistance.

It is extremely important for those who are involved in patient care to realize that if the culture allows free expression of feelings the person in pain will moan and cry without shame or inhibition. This is not necessarily indictive of more intense pain and need not be discouraged. We should be concerned with and treat pain without interfering with the person's right to express what he or she feels.

It is also important to make this distinction when preparing couples for childbirth. The childbirth educator must be extremely careful not to impose her own culturally conditioned standards of acceptable behavior upon her students. To do so would give rise to anxiety about performance and discourage communication about actual sensation (some women feel that if they experience pain, they have somehow "failed").

In the past, childbirth preparation has occasionally been aimed at behavioral control. In actuality, the behavior of the laboring woman (or her use or nonuse of specific techniques) is of far less importance than how she feels about her experience. Interestingly, the new mother remembers *how she felt* during labor more clearly than how she behaved. New parents, in relating their labor experience, frequently disagree; the woman may state that she "lost control" or "panicked," while her husband describes her as having been "magnificently calm." He remembers her actual behavior, while she remembers only her focused tension.

Another cultural variable is in the level of pain acceptance. In the Western world we have been unwilling to accept pain as a part of childbearng, and much research into ways of avoiding or alleviating it has been done. The peoples of some Eastern European countries (Poland, for example) both expect and accept pain in childbirth; therefore, they have given little attention to its possible relief.[9]

Livingston presents a modality for describing the responses to pain that may be applied to childbirth.[5] He refers to the physiological, behavioral, and cognitive dimensions as levels of response. The first and lowest level of response is the physiological or visceral level in which the blood pressure and pulse rises and the person prepares for flight. The next level is the behavorial or muscular level of response when the individual tightens up or withdraws, and the third and highest level is the cognitive level when the stimulus is interpreted and an appropriate response is transmitted. The responses of the woman who is unprepared for childbirth are largely at the physiological and muscular levels, with little in the cognitive level. Prenatal conditioning can prepare her to focus her attention on the organization of directed motor activity so that she responds more in the cognitive level, and her responses will be brought into balance (Fig. 2-4).

Perception

Having defined the pain stimulus and the neurologic, physiological and behavioral responses to it, we are now prepared to turn our attention to the perceptual aspects of pain. Perception is the meaning given to the signals that are received, and previous conditioning is of prime importance, for our perceptions are merely the product of the expectations we have learned from certain stimuli.

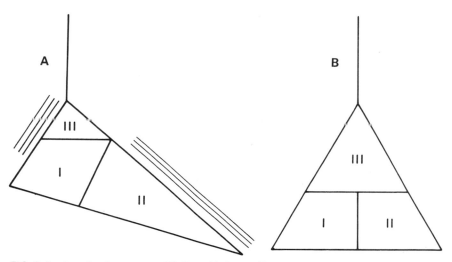

FIG. 2-4. Levels of response. (*A*) Out of balance. Responses largely in physiological (*I*) and muscular or behavioral (*II*) levels. Little response in cognitive (*III*) level. (*B*) In balance. Response largely in cognitive (*III*) level, which organizes and directs muscular (*II*) level (reduced tension, respiratory response) and physiological (*I*) level (reduced pulse, respirations, and blood pressure).

Increase in Perception

The expectations with which the parturient approaches her confinement have a marked effect upon the subjective course of her labor. If she expects to suffer she will surely suffer, even in a perfectly normal and uncomplicated labor.

The universal use of the word *pain* as a synonym for contraction preconditions the expectation that it must be inherently painful, even if the woman has otherwise managed to escape the horrendous tales that surround pregnancy and childbirth. Occasionally one sees the woman in early labor who comes in to be examined because of strange tightenings in her belly. Only when it is identified to her as labor does she begin to perceive it as painful and to exhibit pain responses.

Anxiety

Anxiety can increase pain perception in the same way. Strong fear, by stimulating the sympathetic nervous system, further increases the physiological reactions. It also inhibits the organized modulating action of the gate control mechanism because of central nervous system disorganization.

Fatigue

Heightened perception of pain may also result from physical and mental fatigue. The ability to cope with discomfort and annoyance decreases with exhaustion; the person is no longer as able to accept and integrate further stimulation.

Muscle Tension

The third major cause of increased pain perception is muscular tension. This effect can be graphically demonstrated in the following experiment: sharply pinch the skin on the back of your wrist and notice the sensation. Now make a fist and hold your forearm in strong contraction for 20 to 30 seconds. Repeat the skin pinch and notice the difference in your perception of the stimulus.

Decrease in Perception

Just as pain perception is enhanced by anxiety, fatigue, or muscle tension, it can be inhibited if these influences are minimized. Unwanted pain perception and responses can also be suppressed by focused attention, which functions primarily as a way for the person to control anxiety about the stimulus. As discussed previously, the relationship between anxiety and pain perception is a close one—namely, low anxiety ratio, increased pain tolerance.

Pain in Childbirth

Among the body's normal physiological functions, uterine contraction alone causes pain. Although the physical causes of childbirth pain have not been definitely established, various hypotheses have been presented, including **hypoxia** of the contracted muscle cells (as in angina pectoris); compression of nerve ganglia in the **cervix** and lower uterine segment by the tightly interlocking muscle bundles; stretching of the cervix during dilatation; and stretching of the **perineum.**[1] Each of these elements is a possible cause of the discomfort that is universally ascribed to childbirth, but the translation of discomfort into pain rests not only upon the strength of the signal but also upon psychological conditioning.

Earlier we considered various ways in which attitudes about pain are conditioned by elements in the family and the culture. There are additional myths surrounding childbirth itself that have a bearing on levels of apprehension both related and unrelated to pain.

In the past there was reason enough to fear for the very life of the parturient woman. Infant and maternal mortality were high, and all the efforts of the medical profession had to be directed to the physical safety of mother and child (perhaps it would be more accurate to say mother *or* child, as one sometimes had to be sacrificed for the life of the other). It is not surprising, therefore, that attitudes toward childbirth were influenced by fears of death and loss. Since attitudes toward pain are ordinarily associated with fear of bodily injury, childbirth fears would naturally be enhanced.

Childbirth Preparation

Childbirth preparation does not alter the primary stimulus arising from the laboring uterus. It can only modify the interpretation and perception of the signal that is received.

Factual relevant information about the course of labor and birth reduces anxiety. Uncertainty about how to cope is replaced with specific techniques that may be employed as the need arises. Although various behavorial options are presented, the goal is a mode of behavior that allows the woman to participate in her labor in a way that is meaningful, relatively comfortable, and physiologically sound. Her ability to cope is reinforced throughout her preparation and childbirth by all members of the childbirth team: husband or labor coach, childbirth educator, physician or midwife, and hospital nurse.

The techniques taught for labor fall into three main categories: (1) relaxation techniques, (2) respiratory techniques, and (3) effective expulsion techniques. The deep relaxation prevents undue muscular fatigue and tension, and does not interfere with circulatory function (carrying away the waste products of uterine activity). When executed properly, the respiratory techniques ensure an adequate exchange of gases and prevent either **hyper-** or **hypoventilation.**

Table 2-1. **Effecting the Relay System**

Relay	Action	Rationale
First	Stroking	Sensory input increased
Second	Organized motor response	Descending messages take precedence in cord
Third	Focused attention (concentration on motor response)	Area of inhibition in cortex, less aware of other incoming signals

    The tactile stimulation that is taught as abdominal stroking increases the input on large-diameter nerve fibers carrying impulses to the cord for transmission to the brain, thus helping to block other impulses that may be arriving at the level of the cord simultaneously. This action on the gate control mechanism is enhanced by the increased activity of the cerebral cortex, which is engaged in focused attention upon the behavioral response. Concentration upon respiration, relaxation, and so forth activates the descending nerve fibers, which direct the response and simultaneously take priority in the central nervous system over incoming signals (Table 2-1).

References

1. Hellman ML, Pritchard JA: Williams Obstetrics, 14th ed, p 353. New York, Appleton-Century-Crofts, 1971
2. Kimball CD: Commentary. ICEA Review 4(3):7, 1980
3. Kimball CD, Chang CM, Huang SM et al: Immunoreactive endorphin peptides and prolactin in umbilical vein and maternal blood. Presented at the annual meeting of the Pacific Coast OB/GYN Society, October 1980
4. Lamaze F: Painless Childbirth: The Lamaze Method. Chicago, Henry Regnery, 1970
5. Livingston WK: What is pain? Sci Am 188:59–66, 1953
6. Melzack R, Wall P: Pain mechanisms: A new theory. Science 150:971–978, 1965
7. Oyama T et al: Beta endorphin in obstetric analgesia. Am J Obstet Gynecol 137:613–616, 1980
8. Sternbach RA: Pain: A Psychophysiological Analysis. New York, Academic Press, 1968
9. Zborowski M: Cultural components in responses to pain. Journal of Social Issues 8:16–30, 1952

3

Psychological Analgesia

In this century we are witnessing an unprecedented increase in the demand for knowledge of and preparation for the childbearing event. This is partly due to the breakdown of traditional patterns of behavior and partly a result of the mood of the times. All traditional areas are being questioned, and mass communication has made the public more aware of its options.

The women's movement has had tremendous impact upon women's concept of themselves during childbirth. The traditional passive acceptance that allowed a woman to be totally anesthetized during an important event in her life has given way to a desire to participate herself and to share this event with her mate. As more information is made available to the public about the emotional aspects of childbearing and their effects upon the new family, couples are demanding to participate. Concurrently, the birth rate is dropping, which hastens the implementation of change through increased need on the part of hospitals and physicians to meet consumer demands.

The idea of family-centered maternity care has been around for more than a quarter of a century, but has only recently been implemented to any extent. There has been a change in obstetric practices in the use of medications and anesthesias as we learn more about their effects upon the newborn. This reduction of pharmacologic intervention makes the preparation and cooperation of the **parturient** desirable. As a result, more and more institutions are offering classes and providing the opportunity for expectant parents to participate if they so desire. A few forward-looking institutions are even offering the expectant parents the opportunity to ask for and expect the kind of childbirth experience that they desire (*e.g.*, low lighting, no episiotomy), as long as their desires do not interfere with good obstetric practices.

Historical Overview

The modern childbirth preparation class developed along two distinct lines that arose from two different needs. One need, felt in the early 1900s, was the public health need to teach mothers about hygiene and good health practices. The other was a desire to find a nonpharmacologic means of reducing or eliminating pain in childbirth. Early childbirth preparation classes concentrated in one or the other of these areas, leaving large gaps in total preparation. Although these two kinds of preparation began with quite divergent goals, today's childbirth preparation classes combine the best of each approach and have many more similarities than differences.

Public Health Needs

The first to recognize the need for better prenatal health care information in this country was the American Red Cross, which offered the first class designed to teach mothers hygiene and baby care as early as 1908. The Maternity Center Association in New York, in the belief that good maternity care is the right rather than the privilege of every women, also offered classes to mothers as early as 1919, and in 1930 waged an active radio campaign urging every woman to seek early prenatal care. Today this association is continuing its pioneering efforts by offering not only classes for parents, but also a school for midwives and workshops for professionals interested in family-centered maternity care.

Out of this public health approach grew the type of classes often referred to as general classes in preparation for childbirth. These classes are often offered by institutions, community organizations, or even physicians in private practice. They are almost entirely informational in nature and include the physical changes that occur during pregnancy, parturition, and the pospartum period, as well as information about the newborn and its care. They may also offer some prenatal and postpartum physical fitness exercises, but little emphasis is placed upon ways to cope with the stresses of labor and delivery.

Pain Reduction

The second major consideration that eventually led to the modern childbirth class was the need for a way to cope with pain that would yield a predictable result for large numbers of women. The first really major attempt to deal with this problem by other than chemical means was made in Russia in the early 1900s. The Russians first experimented with hypnosis, but this proved unpredictable and ineffective for large groups. When Erofeeva demonstrated the conditioned character of pain in 1912, the Russians began to explore the concept of deconditioning noxious expectations of childbirth and conditioning a new response.[9] For the first time, the inevitability of pain in childbirth was questioned. Previous methods had approached the problem by attempting to minimize pain; the new method sought to find the cause (no longer believed to be physical in origin) and eradicate it.[14] Because of the stress upon the *prevention* of pain by psychological means, rather than the lessening of pain, the Soviets called their new method **psychoprophylaxis.**

Psychoprophylaxis was observed by the French obstetrician Lamaze while on a trip to the USSR in 1951. He made some changes to suit the less controlled environment of the French culture and began to educate women about pregnancy and childbirth. From this modest beginning, psycho-prophylaxis as a method of childbirth preparation spread rapidly through-out Europe. At about the same time, it was instituted as the approved method for delivery in China. It went virtually unnoticed in the United States until Marjorie Karmel, a mother who had been delivered by the Lamaze method in France, was seeking an obstetrician to deliver her second child in the United States. The story of her search and frustration is recorded in her book, *Thank You, Dr. Lamaze,* which was published in 1959.[6]

Two years later, the American Society of Psychoprophylaxis in Obstetrics, Inc. (ASPO) was founded by seven New York obstetricians. ASPO, which later expanded to include instructors in the psychopro-phylactic method as well as parent members, has as its goal the dissemina-tion of the psychoprophylactic method. Largely through the efforts of ASPO, psychoprophylaxis, or the Lamaze method as it is sometimes called, has become well known and is accepted in most areas of the United States today.

In the 1920s, independent of the Soviet studies, Dick-Read, a lone practitioner in Birmingham, England, was also studying the effects of education upon the amount of pain perceived by women in labor. He had observed the relative ease with which women who expected little or no pain gave birth. He questioned the safety of the **analgesics** then available, and his experience led him to believe that the emotional state in which the woman labored had a major influence upon the subjective outcome.

In 1933 Dick-Read published his book, *Natural Childbirth,* advocat-ing the reduction of fear through education and emotional support. He states that the most important cause of pain in normal childbirth is fear. Using the term *fear–tension–pain syndrome,* he explains how fear alone can interefere with the smooth working of the laboring uterus by the action of the sympathetic nervous system, ". . . creating a condition of rigidity in the lower segment and outlet of the organ . . . ," thus "introducing resistance to the efforts of the longitudinal muscle fibers." In addition, Dick-Read states that tension interferes with circulation to the uterus, allowing the waste products of muscle work to build up, increasing muscle irritability and causing eventual mild anoxia of the uterus with a resultant reduction of efficiency.[4]

Natural childbirth, as Dick-Read called his method, was a tremendous leap toward humanism in the delivery room. Sadly, he did not support his writings with sufficient scientific evidence to convince his colleagues, who had become experts in the use of anesthetics and surgical intervention. His own patients did exceedingly well under his tutelage, but those instructors who followed him had somewhat less predictable results. Despite the excellent work done at Yale and the studies by Thoms, natural childbirth was never completely accepted as a preferred method for coping with the stresses of labor in the majority of Western countries.[12,13]

Methods

Stevens has given us an outline of the strategies used in all methods of psychological pain reduction.[11] They include the following:

1. Systematic relaxation (controlled relaxation)
2. Cognitive control
    a. Disassociation strategies (focusing attention upon some aspect of the stimulus other than pain, *e.g.*, the wavelike character of the contraction)
    b. Interference strategies
       (1) Distraction (useful in early labor)
       (2) Attention focusing (concentration on learned technique)
3. Rehearsal (practicing the desired responses in nonstressful setting, role playing the desired behavior)
4. Support and attention from the childbirth team
5. Desensitization (realistic description of what labor is like, open discussion of fears)

The reader who desires a comprehensive discussion of psychological strategies for diminution of pain in childbirth is referred to Bonica, who has devoted five chapters to this subject in his monumental *Principles and Practice of Obstetric Analgesia and Anesthesia.*[1]

Because the various methods have so strongly influenced each other in the course of their evolvement, it is no simple task to contrast them. All approaches are based upon education and psychological support for the parturient. The differences lie in emphasis and techniques for labor.

Although the psychoprophylactic method and the psychophysical method are the two main approaches to childbirth preparation that are preferred in the United States today, other methods are being taught by some childbirth instructors.

The Psychoprophylactic Method

The psychoprophylactic method (PPM) is a highly structured approach that rests upon a tripod base of conditioning, concentration, and discipline to yield a predictable response. Preparation for labor as a physical event might be compared to the way in which an athlete prepares for an athletic event; the required skill is practiced repetitively so that the body will respond in the desired way. Athletes concentrate all of their effort on improvement until they are conditioned (or "in condition") to perform at their maximum ability. Likewise, the parturient takes an active role in the learning process as well as responsibility for carrying out her tasks in labor.

In addition, a labor coach is prepared to give psychological and physical support. In the United States this coach is usually the expectant father, although another caring person in the woman's life or a hired *monitrice* could fulfill this task if the father is unavailable. Interestingly, as the pregnant woman's need for dependence increases in her final trimester, the person who will be with her in labor assumes a meaningful place in her life even if he or she does not do so at other times.

Conditioning

Conditioning is essential to PPM. A **conditioned response** is defined as one that becomes associated with a previously unrelated stimulus through repeated presentation of the stimulus at the same time with a stimulus normally yielding the response. An example of this behavior is that of an infant who normally salivates when the nipple touches his mouth. Gradually, through repetition of the temporal association, the sight of the bottle or breast causes the infant to salivate before the nipple touches his mouth. The sight stimulus becomes a stimulus for the conditioned response.

Because humans are capable of abstract thought, language can be substituted for the actual stimulus in the conditioning process; thus expectation plays a role. For example, the knowledge that many young people have about childbirth is limited to the fact that labor begins when a woman feels her first "pain." Because of the lack of support, knowledge, and patterning of childbearing behavior, the woman inevitably responds to contractions in the same way she customarily responds to pain: muscular tension, fear, crying out, breath holding. The resultant visceral responses are elevated blood pressure and pulse. The culture in which the woman lives conditioned her to an expectation of pain and thereby a pain response.

Putting the question of pain aside for a moment, this fragmented muscular and visceral response is deleterious to the smooth progression of the labor because it squanders the woman's energies in tension and flight reactions and compromises her respiratory exchange. These considerations alone would make the substitution of a new response desirable.

In PPM classes the parturient is taught to practice behavior during contractions by consciously relaxing and breathing in a precise pattern. The practice is preceded by the verbal cue "contraction begins" and followed by the cue "contraction ends." This use of precise verbal cues helps her to associate her behavioral response (controlled relaxation, respiratory technique) with the contraction, rather than an abstract practice technique. The more faithfully she and her labor coach rehearse in this precise manner, associating the cue with the institution of the behavioral response, the more probable this response becomes for actual labor. Conditioned responses are unstable, however, and if the acquired behavior is not reinforced through intensive practice as confinement approaches they can become less reliable. For this reason, classes in PPM are scheduled to finish close to the expected due date, when motivation is at its peak.

Concentration

Impulses traveling through the central nervous system continuously bombard the cerebral cortex with information about the environment and the internal workings of the body. At any given time, hundreds of such impulses are received, although most do not reach the level of awareness. The signal that is the strongest, or upon which the person has focused his attention, reaches consciousness, while the other signals are diminished. This occurs through the phenomena of excitation and inhibition.[2] The strongest stimulus produces a focus of positive excitation that begins to diffuse throughout the cortex. However, since total takeover by one stimulus would be unsafe for the individual, the surrounding tissue responds with an area of inhibition. This serves to concentrate and contain the area of excitation.

In labor, the strongest signal is that arising from the laboring uterus. The attention of the unprepared woman is focused upon the sensation of the "labor pain" and her fear; she is only minimally aware of offers to assist her or of possible comfort measures. It is as if she withdraws into her misery. PPM proposes to substitute a stronger area of excitation through concentration upon the execution of the behavioral response. Thus the onset of the contraction becomes a signal to use the body in a precise learned way which the woman and her coach have practiced intensively in the prenatal period. It is her active concentration, focused upon execution of motor skills, that reinforces the strength of the area of inhibition and minimizes the awareness of other sensations. This directed activity takes precedence over fragmented random responses for as long as equilibrium can be maintained.

Discipline

Discipline is required to practice the techniques over and over again in the preparatory period, using the verbal cues ("contraction begins, contraction ends") and tactile cues (stroking to signal release of muscle tension), so that conditioning can take place. The woman and her coach must discipline themselves to practice their roles repetitively so that they can maintain equilibrium by adapting to changing needs during the course of labor. If the woman does not personally accept the responsibility of controlling her responses in labor, the entire structure falls apart.

The possibility of remaining in control of behavioral responses, giving the illusion of being in control of the environment, appeals to many. PPM implements the integration of responses by providing a specific way to respond to the contractions. The responses allow the woman to see herself as someone who is able to cope, which in turn reinforces the probability of continued coping behavior (Fig. 3–1).

If the woman loses control, however, this behavior too will reinforce itself; she sees herself in such distress that she can no longer direct her behavior. Her behavior becomes fragmented, with a marked increase in anxiety as well as muscular and visceral responses. Immediate intervention is indicated to help the woman regain her self-possession.

The labor coach has been specifically prepared for this possibility. Because the couple has used the discipline of repeated practice in a precise structured manner, the reinstitution of the verbal and tactile cues should elicit a conditioned response. The coach immediately reinforces this response by making positive comments and giving encouragement. In addition, the coach may provide a model by maintaining eye contact with the parturient and doing the breathing with her for a few contractions until she feels able to continue.

If this is not enough to allow the woman to regain her equilibrium, pharmacologic agents may augment the effects of PPM. Medications used judiciously are not contraindicated when the need exists. In childbirth classes the instructor should stress the need for good communication between parturient and physician or midwife so that each knows what the

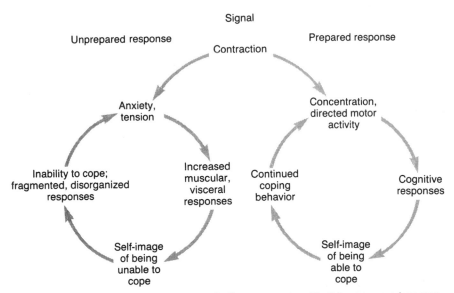

FIG. 3–1. The continuum of responses in the prepared and in the unprepared woman.

other expects in labor and delivery. Thus, the woman need not fear that she will be "knocked out" if she accepts medication. The decision to accept or to ask for medication should be a result of knowledge and informed consent.

Childbirth Without Pain

The Childbirth Without Pain Education Association of Detroit was founded by Flora Hommel, a nurse who observed psychoprophylaxis in France and studied with Lamaze. This organization has retained the original emphasis upon painlessness in childbirth because its proponents feel (along with French practitioners of *accouchement sans douleur*) that if a woman "expects to feel pain, she will feel it, no matter what the sensation is really."[12] Hommel writes that she believes women are drawn to PPM for Painless Childbirth programs precisely because of the title. After attending classes, most find that their "values change and goals broaden."[5] Other than the emphasis upon painlessness as a goal, PPM is presented as previously discussed.

The New Childbirth

In association with the National Childbirth Trust in England, Wright and Phillip have developed a method based upon psychoprophylactic preparation, which they call "the new childbirth." The breathing techniques for labor are similar to those of PPM (see Appendix A), but are presented somewhat differently.[15] They are described as "levels of breathing" in the sense of shifting gears from first to second to third and back again as more concentration is needed.

Psychophysical Preparation

The psychophysical approach to childbirth is less structured in content and presentation than PPM. Like PPM, it is based upon education about childbearing to relieve anxiety generated by misinformation, and strong psychological support for the parturient by other members of the childbirth team.

Because Dick-Read's "natural childbirth" relies upon the individual woman's body to tell her how to breathe or react, the techniques were never fully developed as a method. Individual instructors made changes according to their own beliefs. An outgrowth of Dick-Read's work, psychophysical preparation is often called "modified Read." It stresses working in harmony with the mechanisms of labor by relaxing and submitting to the body's demands, breathing more rapidly and deeply as the strength of the contraction increases to ensure an adequate respiratory exchange.

Although some women have been able to remain comfortable throughout labor by simple relaxation, many find this role too passive in spite of strong support from helpers. Possibly due to the fact that women are encouraged to withdraw into themselves, they become less aware of support from those around them.

Because classes are unstructured, discussion techniques are the primary teaching tool in psychophysical classes. Proponents of this approach believe that true undirected agenda gathering (from the group) most nearly meets the needs of the learners. Respiratory and relaxation techniques are taught as a possible help to interrupt the fear–tension–pain cycle in labor. By teaching techniques for labor in this nondirective way, psychophysical instructors feel that use or nonuse of techniques can be decided upon at the time of labor. This encourages freedom of choice and implies responsibility for the choice without the bias inherent in the conditioning process of PPM.

The Bradley Method

The Bradley approach to childbearing grew concurrently with PPM in the United States, and uses many similar techniques. However, it does not rely upon concentration and conditioning, but stresses working in harmony with the body.

Bradley, a Denver obstetrician, observed the ease with which animals give birth and drew some correlations with human birth. The techniques that he advocates for physical conditioning and for labor are drawn from these observations and adapted to the human bipedal posture. Bradley feels that women can give birth in a truly natural way, that is, in a way more closely allied to the laws of nature without the noxious influence of cultural conditioning.

Bradley does an excellent job of explaining the rationale for the various physical fitness exercises, which he divides into "the three Bs"— back, bottom, belly. For example, it is recommended that pelvic rocking on hands and knees be done vigorously each night to bring the uterus up and forward, more nearly the position it would hold if the woman were still a quadruped. This not only increases flexibility in the lower back, but reduces pressure on the pelvic area and on vessels returning blood from the lower extremities. The woman should then go directly to bed, being sure to lie on her side so that the weight of the baby is supported by the bed.

Bradley method teachers believe that true natural childbirth can and will take place in normal births if the expectant mother and father are properly prepared for the labor experience. They are strongly opposed to any form of anesthesia or **analgesia** because of the effects upon the fetus and claim a 94% medication-free success rate. (Their teachers must maintain this high rate of medication-free deliveries to maintain their certification with the American Academy of Husband Coached Childbirth.)

For labor, complete deep relaxation is the main technique. The husband observes his wife during sleep to learn her natural sleep position because this position is the one most comfortable for her and will be used during labor. In class he is taught to signal relaxation by stroking and verbalizing in ways that are best for them. For example, he might use endearments or relate a narrative of pleasant times past for his wife to recall. He helps her to disassociate from the present and create a serene frame of mind. He may say, "During the contractions we will do this . . . " to rehearse the labor situation, but does not use the precise verbal cues used in PPM.

The breathing used for labor, because Bradley believes it should be a natural type of breathing, is a deep diaphragmatic type which is normally used in sleep. The husband/coach is instructed again to observe how his wife breathes when deeply asleep, because this is the breathing pattern she should use for labor.[3]

Psychosexual Preparation

In the psychosexual approach, childbirth is considered "a part of the very wide spectrum of sexuality in a woman's life ranging all the way from her image of herself as a woman, through making love and the processes of childbearing . . . her reactions to menstruation and the menopause."[7] Developed in England by Kitzinger, it is based upon Dick-Read's earlier work. Exercises are therefore described in terms of physiological processes and working in harmony with the body.

Kitzinger drew upon her background in dramatics, anthropology, and counseling to create a method that uses the body's sensory memory of past sensation, imagery, and tactile cues. For example, the feeling of unzipping a tight girdle is suggested for general torso relaxation, or the image of a dress slipping off a hanger is evoked to bring about relaxation of the shoulders. The student is instructed to relax more on each exhalation as she imagines the dress slipping, slipping from its hanger. In this way, she learns to relax consciously on each exhalation as she needs to do in labor. Tactile cues for relaxation are equally important, with the woman relaxing "toward" her husband's hand. During labor he strokes areas of tension to enhance relaxation as well as to make a caring gesture.

The woman's ability to control the muscles of the perineum and birth canal is given special attention. After being taught the importance of control both for lovemaking and for voluntary release of the muscles during delivery, the woman is taught to differentiate between the various muscles (pubococcygeus, levator ani, gluteal muscles, adductors of the thighs), alternately tensing and releasing them singly, then in association.[8] Finally, she is taught to associate the perineal area, which is under stress during labor and therefore inclined to become tense, with the jaw, which is not under stress at that time. The relaxation of the jaw is linked with the relaxation of the perineum on the theory that when the parturient is smiling, jaw relaxed, by association she allows the perineum to relax.

Because Kitzinger views pregnancy as only a part of the whole psychosexual life cycle, including the woman's relationship with her husband, parents, and children, marriage counseling in private sessions is included as a part of her method.

Birth Without Violence

Birth Without Violence is not a method of preparation for birth at all, but is included here because of the numerous questions concerning it. LeBoyer, who developed this method of delivery in France, is a strong advocate of the infant. He empathizes with the infant undergoing the trauma of birth, being born into cold, bright, noisy surroundings and being suspended unsupported by its ankles. LeBoyer advocates diminished sound and light in the delivery room, late clamping of the cord, warm room temperature, and a warm bath so that the newborn can become accustomed gradually to its new environment. In addition, the newborn is placed on the mother's stomach and gently massaged until the **placenta** detaches.

Birth without violence is finding rapid acceptance among the public, but testing has not yet been adequate to establish if infants delivered in this way are indeed calmer and more serene from the start than infants who are held gently, dried off, and handed to their parents. Although many feel that LeBoyer overstates his case in *Birth Without Violence,* he has raised many questions about how delivery room practices may affect the newborn infant.[10]

References

1. Bonica JJ: Principles and Practice of Obstetric Analgesia and Anesthesia, Vols I and II. Philadelphia, FA Davis, 1969
2. Bonstein I: Painless Childbirth, pp 23–25. London, William Heinemann, 1958
3. Bradley R: Husband Coached Childbirth, p 74. New York, Harper & Row, 1965
4. Dick-Read G: Childbirth Without Fear, pp 61, 62. New York, Harper & Row, 1970
5. Hommel F: Painless? Childbirth. Childbirth Education, (Journal of the American Society of Psychoprophylaxis in Obstetrics) 2:4, 1969
6. Karmel M: Thank You, Dr. Lamaze. Philadelphia, J B Lippincott, 1959
7. Kitzinger S: The Experience of Childbirth. Middlesex, England, Pelican Books, 1970
8. Kitzinger S: Giving Birth. New York, Taplinger, 1971
9. Lamaze F: Painless Childbirth: The Lamaze Method. a, p 33; b, p 12. Chicago, Henry Regnery, 1970

10. LeBoyer F: Birth Without Violence. New York, Alfred Knopf, 1975
11. Stevens R: Psychological strategies for management of pain in prepared childbirth. Presented at ICEA Convention, Seattle, Washington, June 16, 1976
12. Thoms H: Implementation of a preparation for parenthood program. Obstet Gynecol 11:593, 1958
13. Thoms H, Karlowsky E: Two thousand deliveries under a training for childbirth program. Am J Obstet Gynecol 68:279, 1954
14. Velvovsky I, Platonov K, Ploticher V, Shugom E: Painless Childbirth Through Psychoprophylaxis. Moscow, Foreign Languages Publishing House, 1960
15. Wright E: The New Childbirth. New York, Hart, 1966

4

Pharmacologic Analgesia
and Anesthesia

The purpose of the childbirth educator is not to give a detailed description of all possible medications and anesthetics that might be employed for labor or delivery, but rather to present an overview of the information that expectant parents need to familiarize themselves with the broad aspects of **analgesia** and anesthesia. The parents come to class with preconceived ideas about medication, some of which result from increased public awareness of the effects of obstetric medication upon the newborn.[2] The instructor should present the benefits of various options without minimizing the hazards involved so that the couple can decide for themselves what they desire. This must be done in a way that relieves anxiety and encourages communication betweeen the couple and their obstetrician or midwife. The parturient should discuss her preferences with her obstetrician so that they can function as a team. Hopsital medication policies also need to be explored, because some hospitals do not allow couples to remain together if the woman receives medication.

The childbirth teacher has a delicate task. On the one hand, she feels she should strongly encourage her students to make complete use of the techniques they have learned to reduce discomfort in labor; on the other, she wants to emphasize the importance of remaining flexible in the use or nonuse of medication so that, should the parturient need medication in addition to her respiratory and relaxation techniques, she will not feel guilty.[4]

The parturient can be given some guidelines so that she can decide whether to ask for or accept medication, and she should be aware that occasionally unforseen circumstances do arise that necessitate intervention. For example, if she feels unable to cope with contractions at 4 cm **dilatation**, she may need medication because she will be having several more hours of labor. If, however, she feels this way at 8 cm dilatation, perhaps the knowledge that the end is near coupled with strong support will be sufficient to get her through the difficult end of the first stage of labor. Students should be reassured that their efforts to cope with pain by learned techniques will greatly reduce, if not eliminate, the need for pharmacologic intervention. Medication, when needed, will be in the minimal amount necessary to deal with residual pain.

Unless a special class is to be set aside to discuss medications and anesthetics, which may place too strong an emphasis on the subject in a six-class series, it seems logical to divide the topic roughly into medications for use during the first stage of labor (analgesics, tranquilizers, sedatives, and amnesics) and those for delivery (anesthetics). Thus, the discussion of analgesics falls into the class about active labor or variations of the first stage, with anesthetics being grouped with delivery and variations of the second stage.

In choosing an appropriate drug for use during labor, the obstetrician must consider the effects upon the labor itself as well as upon the mother and fetus. Medication administered too early, or in large doses, may occasionally prolong the labor process.

Studies have show that the fetus is affected by all medications administered to the mother and Brazelton has stated that the "effects of any perceptible amount of medication administered during labor are evident in the newborn for at least a week."[1,2] Other researchers have felt that the newborn's responses are retarded for an even longer period.[1] Even if the infant is quickly resuscitated at delivery, his immature liver is incapable of immediately metabolizing the narcotic remaining in his system. The sucking and gag reflexes, so necessary for survival, are therefore compromised by the remaining narcotic. In addition, there are implications for early parent–child interaction when the infant is lethargic and unresponsive to the new parent's efforts to feed and care for him.[2]

Medications for the First Stage of Labor

The terms used in parents' classes should be those they may hear used in the hospital. Commonly, the term *medication* refers to analgesics and tranquilizers; terms such as *painkiller* should be avoided because they have a negative connotation.

Analgesics

An analgesic agent is one whose primary function is to relieve pain. Examples of the analgesics most commonly seen in the labor room are meperidine hydrochloride (Demerol) and alphaprodine hydrochloride (Nisentil). When given in small doses, these agents may prove helpful to the parturient who cannot quite cope with her contractions. They may help her to relax and raise her tolerance for pain so that she can continue to use her techniques. When given, they reach a peak of effectiveness in about 60 to 90 minutes and last for about 2 to 3 hours. However, they are central nervous system depressants and readily cross the placenta, affecting the fetus. Moya and Thorndike have given parameters for minimal narcotic effect on the infant of more than 6 hours prior to delivery or less than 1 hour (Table 4-1).[5]

Tranquilizers

Since the amount of narcotic necessary to reduce pain in a particular person has a direct relationship to the amount of anxiety present, the obstetrician sometimes orders a tranquilizer to reduce the narcotic dosage necessary. Tranquilizers are of low molecular weight and therefore cross the placenta readily. However, studies have not shown that these drugs affect the **Apgar rating** of the infants studied.[3] The most commonly used tranquilizers are promethazine hydrochloride (Phenergan), propiomazine hydrochloride (Largon), hydroxyzine hydrochloride (Vistaril), and diazepam (Valium).

Sedatives

Sedatives, such as the barbiturates, are occasionally used in early labor to induce sleep. For example, if a woman in very early labor arrives at the hospital after a long night of timing contractions, she is already fatigued and assumes that she must be in advanced labor because she has been timing contractions for so long. The physician may order a barbiturate in order to allow this woman a few hours sleep so that she will be refreshed before she goes into advanced labor.

The barbiturates have a prolonged action and a slow rate of metabolism, however, meaning that effects may be noted in mother and infant for a long time after the dose is given. In addition, barbiturates may make the parturient uncooperative and irritable if the labor progresses before she has had the chance for adequate rest.

Amnesics

In the unprepared woman the amnesic known as scopolamine is sometimes used for the first stage of labor to cause the woman to forget her labor.

In the traditional delivery of a generation ago, scopolamine was combined with large doses of barbiturates and meperidine, and administered every several hours. The effects were delirium and amnesia. The women were often tied down in criblike cages for their own protection; they were unable to cooperate or understand. True, for many there was a complete memory gap when they groggily awoke several hours later, but the memory of fear and focused tension often remained. Scopolamine is to be strongly discouraged for the prepared woman if she has any desire to participate in the birth.

(Text continues on p 44)

Table 4-1. **Effects of Agents Used for Pain Relief During labor**

Agent or Technique	Optimal Dose	Therapeutic Effect	Maternal Side-Effect	Fetal/Newborn Side-Effect	Miscellaneous Information
Sedatives					
Secobarbital (Seconal) Pentobarbital (Nembutal)	100 mg IM, 50 mg IV 100 mg IM, PO, 50 mg IV	Sedation and sleep	Vertigo, decreased perception of sensory stimuli, nausea and vomiting, decreased blood pressure	Possible central nervous system depression or apnea	May cause restlessness when used alone; may slow labor
Phenobarbital (Luminal)	100 mg IV, PO				
Tranquilizers					
Diazepam (Valium)	2, 5 or 10 mg IV, IM, PO	Lowered tension and apprehension levels	Vertigo, drowsiness, decreased blood pressure	Possible CNS depression	Enhances analgesic drug action
Hydroxyzine (Vistaril) Propiomazine (Largon) Promethazine (Phenergan) Promazine (Sparine)	5–15 mg IM, PO 20–40 mg IM, PO 25–50 mg IM, PO 25 mg IM, PO				
Analgesics					
Meperidine (Demerol) Morphine sulfate Alphaprodine (Nisentil)	50–100 mg IM 8–15 mg IM 20–40 mg IM, IV	Increased pain threshhold	Nausa and vomiting, mild respiratory and circulatory depression	Possible CNS depression	Not given when delivery imminent; used in combination with tranquilizers
General Anesthetics					
Trichloroethylene (Trilene) Methoxyflurane (Penthrane) Nitrous Oxide Cyclopropane	0.5 % 0.3–0.5 % 40 % 3–5 % (inhalation)	Analgesia during 1st stage of labor; loss of consciousness in 2nd stage	Possible aspiration or cyanosis	Possible CNS depression or hypoxia	Trilene volatile; Trilene and Penthrane can be self-administered by hand-held mask
Diethyl ether Halothane	2–5 % 0.5–1 %				

Local anesthetics
Procaine (Novocain)
Dibucaine (Nupercaine)
Lidocaine (Xylocaine)
Tetracaine (Pontocaine)
Mepivacaine (Carbocaine)
Chloroprocaine (Nesacaine)
Bupivacaine (Marcaine)

Types of local analgesia

	Concentration varies from 0.5–2 % solutions	Loss of sensation by blocking conduction of nerve impulses	Effects depend on mode of administration	Effects depend on mode of administration	Effects depend on mode of administration
Epidural block Caudal block	5–15 ml of 1, 1.5, or 2% solutions	High degree of pain relief	Mild hypotension is frequent; loss of bearing-down reflex in 2nd stage	None unless severe sustained maternal hypotension	May slow labor; epidural blocks pain at each stage of labor; caudal causes mild hypotension
Paracervical block	5–10 ml of 1% solution bilaterally	Temporary block of pain during labor	Transient depression of contractions	Occasional bradycardia	Analgesia during labor; but no perineal anesthesia
Pudendal block	5–10 ml of 1% solution bilaterally	Nerve block for 2nd stage of labor	Loss of bearing-down reflex	Rarely any	Does not relieve contraction pain, anesthetizes perineum
Saddle block	1–1.5 ml concentration depends on agent used	High degree of pain relief	Occasionally, postspinal headache	Rarely any	Uncomfortable position while block administered; can be used only when delivery is imminent; excellent for delivery

Grad R. Woodside J: Obstetrical analgesics and anesthesia. Am J Nurs 73:243, 1977.
Copyright February 1977, the American Journal of Nursing Company. Reproduced with permission.

Anesthesia

Unlike an analgesic, which relieves pain, an anesthetic agent eliminates sensation, either by removing the mother from consciousness or by interrupting the conduction of nerve impulses through the central nervous system. It is important for the childbirth educator to give a broad idea of what the differences between anesthetics are, how they feel, how they are administered, how they affect the baby, and what the risks and benefits are. Even if a particular anesthetic is not one of choice for the prepared woman, it should be included in the class discussion.

Inhalation Anesthesia

The prepared woman would not expect to have a general anesthetic during the birth of her child. However, the instructor should not condemn the general anesthetic, as it is sometimes necessary if an emergency such as prolapse of the umbilical cord requires that the woman be quickly anesthetized and delivered. Put into this framework, "for the good of the infant," most parents would not fight its use for genuine emergencies. If general anesthesia is indicated, it is often combined with a **pudendal block** so that the level of anesthesia may be as light as possible for the sake of the infant.[3]

The drawbacks of general anesthesia are its effects upon the infant, including possible central nervous system depression or hypoxia, and the fact that the mother is removed from awareness at a most important event in her psychosexual life.

Conduction Anesthesia

The Novocain- or xylocaine-like anesthetics used for conduction anesthesia do not affect the fetus directly unless they inadvertently enter the circulatory system. Indirect effects, for example, impairment of fetomaternal circulation and anoxia in the fetus, may be noted if the mother becomes hypotensive, as is sometimes the case when regional anesthesia causes large-scale vasodilatation of the lower extremities. The supine position aggravates this possibility because the venous return is then impeded by the weight of the uterine contents pressing down upon the inferior vena cava. See Table 4-2 for methods and uses of conduction anesthesia.

Local Anesthesia

Local infiltration anesthesia is the direct injection of an anesthetic agent into the area of discomfort. The most common use of this type of anesthetic is injection into the tissues surrounding the perineum for the

Table 4-2. Conduction Anesthesia in Labor: Methods and Uses

Source of Discomfort	Pathways	Relieved by	Comments
Early first stage			
Dilatation of cervix and contraction of body of uterus	Sympathetic nerves to lumbar and thoracic sympathetic chain	Paravertebral block; lumbar sympathetic block; low dose epidural; rhythmic chest breathing	Prepared childbirth techniques very effective; minimal effect on baby; administered in labor room
Late first stage			
Dilatation of cervix approaching transition	Sympathetic nerves to lumbar and thoracic sympathetic chain	Above plus paracervical block, shallow breathing or combined rhythm	Given at 5-6 cm in labor room; occasional fetal bradycardia, depending on dose and local anesthetic used
Early second stage			
Distention of the lower birth canal	Conveyed by pudendal nerves	Caudal epidural; lumbar epidural (higher dose)	Anesthetic given around dura; effective through delivery when catheter used; some hypotension, alteration of contraction and fetal problems depending on dose, placement and agent
		Pudendal block	Given by obstetrician in delivery room; contractions not impaired; patient able to push if alert and coached
Late second stage			
	Conveyed by pudendal nerves	Above plus spinal anesthesia; expulsion techniques	Given on side or sitting position in delivery room just prior to delivery; immediate onset; true saddle experiences contractions; spinal unable to push effectively combined with forceps; hypotension, spinal headache 7-10%

From the outline developed by Dr. Robert Schuder, from the presentation given at the Annual Symposium of Council of Childbirth Education Specialists, Inc, Tarrytown, New York, November 1, 1975. Used with permission.

episiotomy. The mother is in delivery position and is probably only minimally aware of the injections being given because these tissues are distended immediately preceding the delivery, and the descent of the baby exerts direct pressure upon the nerves. The numbing effects of the anesthetic agent will have taken effect by the time the **episiotomy** is repaired.

The mother should be aware that she will experience a pulling sensation as the episiotomy is being repaired. If she is anxious about this, she may be coached to use her controlled relaxation technique again. However, simple distraction by handing her the newborn is usually sufficient.

Regional Anesthesia

Regional anesthetics are injected either into the nerve plexus or around sympathetic nerve pathways to block impulses leading from the uterus by way of the uterosacral and broad ligaments to the cord.[3] A common example that may be useful in class is that of the regional anesthetic used in dentistry; nearly everyone has felt how an injection into the nerve plexus (trigeminal) numbs the entire cheek, lip, and part of the tongue as well as the area being worked on.

Local anesthetic may be injected paracervically either at 3:00 and 9:00 or uterosacrally at 4:00 and 8:00 (Fig. 4-1, *A*). This **paracervical block** may be used during the late first stage if speedy cervical dilatation is desired. It is effective for about 60 to 90 minutes. Drawbacks include occasional fetal **bradycardia,** possibly due to the anesthetic being absorbed by or inadvertently injected into the uterine vessels.

The *pudendal block* is used to relieve pain in the vaginal and perineal area for the second stage of labor and delivery. It should be administered about 30 minutes prior to delivery for maximum effectiveness. It may be used effectively in the prepared woman for **forceps** and breech deliveries, in which her pushing efforts are especially helpful to minimize the amount of pull with the forceps required to effect the delivery (Fig. 4-1, *B*). The anesthetic may be administered either through the vagina, as illustrated, or through the buttock.

As with the local anesthetic, the parturient needs to be forewarned that, even though she is numbed, she will feel the sensation of tissue manipulation as the episiotomy is being repaired and the postpartum vaginal inspection is being carried out. Her conscious relaxation is important, and she may return to her rhythmic breathing pattern and controlled relaxation if necessary.

Extradural Anesthesia

Extradural anesthesia is produced by the injection of a local anesthetic into the extradural space. It differs from a spinal in that the medication

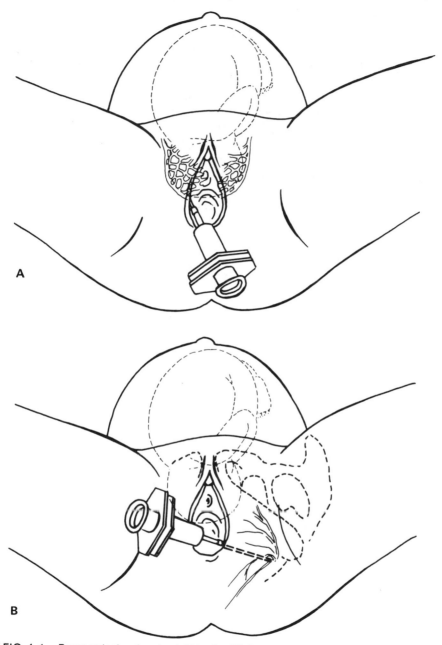

FIG. 4-1.   Paracervical and pudendal blocks. (A) Paracervical block. Sensation from the uterus is carried by way of the broad and uterosacral ligaments. Blocking the sympathetic pathways anywhere between the cervix and the spinal cord is effective in relieving pain in the first stage of labor. (B) Pudendal block, which relieves pain in the vaginal and perineal area, is useful during the second and third stages, including postpartum vaginal inspection and episiotomy repair. (Ross Clinical Education Aid No. 17, Regional Anesthesia in Obstetrics. Columbus, Ross Laboratories, 1968)

neither enters the cord nor mixes with spinal fluid but exerts its influence on the nerve trunks distal to the dura. One way of explaining the difference to parents is to suggest that the medication bathes the membrane surrounding the cord to produce the anesthetic effects. **Caudal** and **epidural** or peridural anesthesias are both included in this group. They differ in site of injection and level of anesthesia that may be obtained.

Continuous forms of these anesthetics may be used for advanced labor in the unprepared woman or for delivery of the prepared woman in the event of obstetric difficulty. The anesthetic is introduced by means of a polyethylene catheter, and the dose may be repeated as needed (Fig. 4-2). This method has the advantage of allowing for lower, more frequent doses. Another advantage of the continuous caudal for labor is that it is pleasant for the parturient. She is free of the stress and discomfort of labor while remaining alert to her surroundings.

There are also disadvantages, however. **Hypotension** may result, labor may be prolonged (especially if it is not well advanced when anesthesia is begun), and the incidence of forceps intervention is greatly increased because the parturient cannot push effectively. This type of anesthesia may

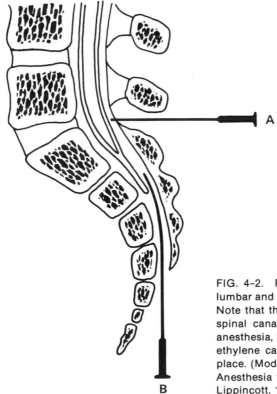

FIG. 4-2. Placement of the needle for (A) lumbar and (B) caudal extradural anesthesia. Note that the needle does not penetrate the spinal canal. For continuous forms of this anesthesia, the needle is replaced by a polyethylene catheter, which is then taped into place. (Modified from Hingson R, Hellman L: Anesthesia for Obstetrics. Philadelphia, J B Lippincott, 1956)

not be an option at smaller hospitals because it requires an anesthetist skilled in its technique. Because continued monitoring by the anesthetist is necessary, it may also be a fairly expensive mode of anesthesia.

Spinal and Saddle Block Anesthesia

The **saddle block** may be the anesthesia of choice for the unprepared woman who prefers to be awake for delivery, especially if extradural anesthesia is unavailable to her. The saddle block is a low spinal, that is, the anesthetic is administered into the spinal canal. The anesthetized area includes those parts of the body that would touch the saddle in horseback riding, as well as the vagina and perineum (Fig. 4–3). The saddle block cannot be given until the cervix is nearly 10 cm dilated to prevent interference with the labor process. Because the woman is unable to push, forceps delivery is mandatory.

The disadvantages include the possibility of hypotension with all of its inherent dangers and the occasional postspinal headache.

Cesarean Sections. Spinal anesthetics are administered into the spinal canal primarily for cesarean sections. The spinal differs from saddle block anesthesia in the level of anesthesia, which reaches well above the umbilicus in a spinal (see Fig. 4–3). Hazards to the fetus are minimized because, unlike inhalation anesthetics, the anesthetic does not enter the circulatory system.

The mother receives the medication curled up on her side and rapidly loses all sensation below the level of the anesthetic. If she is to remain awake during the birth, she needs to be reassured that she will be screened so that she (and her coach, if the modern family centered approach is allowed) will

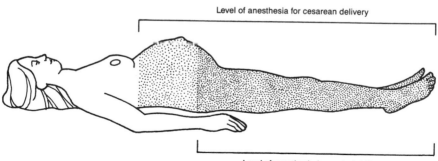

Level of anesthesia for cesarean delivery

Level of anesthesia for vaginal delivery

FIG. 4–3. Levels of anesthesia for cesarean or vaginal delivery. The level of anesthesia for vaginal delivery includes the pelvic area, perineum, and legs. Anesthesia may be either extradural (epidural or caudal) or intraspinal (saddle block). For cesarean delivery, in which abdominal relaxation is necessary, the level of anesthesia includes the above, plus the suprapubic and abdominal areas. Anesthesia may be extradural or spinal. (Modified from Ross Clinical Education Aid No. 17, Regional Anesthesia in Obstetrics. Columbus, Ross Laboratories, 1968)

not be looking directly into the incision. Also, she should be prepared for the sensation of tissue manipulation, which may be described as a tugging sensation. The anesthetist seated at the head monitoring her responses will keep her informed, and she will be able to hear her child's first cry and to see it immediately after the delivery.

References

1. Bowes WA, Brackbill Y, Conway E, Steinschneider AJ: The effects of obstetrical medication on fetus and infant. Monogr Soc Res Child Dev (Serial # 137) 35:4, 1970
2. Brazelton TB: What Childbirth Drugs Can Do to Your Child. Redbook Magazine, Feb 1971
3. Flowers C: Obstetric Analgesia and Anesthesia. New York, Harper & Row, 1967
4. Hingson R, Hellman L: Anesthesia for Obstetrics. Philadelphia, J B Lippincott, 1956
5. Moya F, Thorndike V: Passage of drugs across the placenta. Am J Obstet Gynecol 84:1778–1798, 1962
6. Schuder RJ: Anesthesia for Obstetrics. Proceeding of the Annual Symposium of Council of Childbirth Education Specialists Inc. Tarrytown, New York, November 1, 1975

5

Pregnancy Classes

Introducing the First and Second Trimesters

The childbirth educator who is planning a class for those in early pregnancy should consider the state of mind of these expectant parents. They are struggling with ambivalence and, if the child is their first, doubts about their changing roles. They must accept the reality of the pregnancy first, then that of the forthcoming infant.

Although many childbirth programs do not accept students until their last trimester, classes early in the childbearing cycle can make the pregnancy go more smoothly by helping the expectant parents anticipate the stresses to come. In these classes, the couple learns about pregnancy; focusing on the immediate helps them in their task of acceptance. Preparation for labor and birth takes place in the final trimester, but in the early months the woman is barely accustomed to the idea of being pregnant. Until the pregnancy begins to "show," it lacks reality. As changes in body shape make it obvious, and when **quickening** takes place, the woman fantasizes about the coming infant and herself in her mothering role (see Childbirth: A Time of Crisis, Chap. 1). At this point the mother is exceptionally open to learning, and we can take advantage of this to teach about the remainder of the pregnancy and planning for parenthood.

The precise material included will vary according to the demands of the group and the time allotted. However, there are several general areas of concern that should be discussed: anatomy and physiology, to explain what is happening within the body; common symptoms of pregnancy, to reduce anxiety; nutrition, to give the mother an awareness of the nutritional needs for optimal baby building; physical fitness and body mechanics, to help her use her body efficiently during pregnancy, and improve muscle tone and circulation. Also, discussions of the newborn, what it is like to be a parent, and what the perinatal period is apt to be like can begin. This is an excellent time to recommend books about parenting, some of which are listed in Appendix C. Although it may seem more logical to discuss parenting after labor and delivery, this is not so. In the final weeks the parents are primarily concerned with the labor and delivery, so much so that other topics receive only secondary attention.

Finally, although it is wise for the childbirth educator to organize her

51

thoughts in a general way about areas to cover, it is essential to be flexible about content in order to remain open to the needs of the particular group.

The following discussion is not meant to be a complete review. It is assumed that the childbirth educator has a basic grounding in obstetrics. The discussion here concerns itself with the kinds of things parents want to know.

An understanding of how the long months of pregnancy prepare the woman's body to give birth is reassuring. The symptoms of pregnancy, such as frequency of urination, fatigue, bleeding gums, nausea, mood swings, leg cramps, and tender breasts can all be put into perspective by an explanation of the causes and a sharing of concern with other class members. If others in the class can offer suggestions and comfort measures (rather than the instructor), it helps to foster the supportive milieu, which is one of the goals of prepared childbirth. The instructor then functions as a resource person, actively offering advice only when called upon or when the class is faced with misinformation. Her role is primarily to strengthen coping mechanisms by letting the students know that their own suggestions are worthwhile.

Anatomy and Physiology

An explanation of anatomy and physiology provides a matrix of information upon which to build the discussion. The external and internal genitalia can be pointed out on charts. Correct terminology should be used to help orient the students to medical terminology and to begin the process of demystifying the whole childbirth experience.

The relationships between the various pelvic organs can be demonstrated on charts while the changes that pregnancy brings about are discussed. The group members should be asked to contribute their own experiences with pregnancy and encouraged to join in the active learning process.

The menstrual cycle is a mystery to many. It is probably not necessary to go into great detail about the interactions of progesterone and estrogen, but it is helpful to summarize the process of conception in words that are meaningful to the learner group. Throughout, the instructor should be careful to allow for questions and to encourage participation of the class.

The following is an example of the kind of information helpful to parents. (Illustrations from the *Birth Atlas*, available from Maternity Center Association, may be helpful [see Appendix C]).

> The uterus is a hollow muscular sac in which the baby grows. The lower third hangs down into the vagina and is called the cervix. The upper part is called the fundus. As you can see from the picture, it is pear shaped and has two narrow tubes, which end in a kind of trumpet-shaped opening, leading from the top. These tubes are called fallopian tubes. Slung underneath the tubes are the ovaries where the female egg cells come from.

Each baby girl is born with literally thousands of immature egg cells, waiting to ripen until she reaches the time of her first period. When she reaches about 12 or 13, stimulated by the hormones of her body, these egg cells (or ova) begin to ripen and are thrown off at the rate of usually one per month.

After being released, the ovum travels from the ovary through the tube for about 5-7 days. It is propelled by the wavelike motion of the tube itself and also by the motion of tiny hairlike cells within the tube. If conception has not taken place within 8 hours of its release from the ovary, the opportunity has been missed for that month. The ovum is then sloughed off with the next period.

The lining of the uterus renews itself each month to make ready for a possible pregnancy. It becomes very soft and succulent, high in blood sugars, receptive. This process begins immediately after the menstrual period. About 14 days before the next period, as the ovum enters the tube, the uterus is nearly ready. About a week before the period, the uterus is ready to receive the conceptus. If conception has not taken place, the uterus sheds its lining as the menstrual flow. This has sometimes been called the "cry of the disappointed uterus." Immediately following, the uterus again begins to make ready for a possible pregnancy, and so the cycle repeats itself.

Sexual intercourse must take place during the receptive time of the month if there is to be a pregnancy. The sperm, which is the name of the cell from the father's penis, is deposited in the vagina but swims vigorously up through the uterus and into the tube where conception takes place (Fig. 5-1). Once the sperm joins the mother's ovum, conception has taken place.

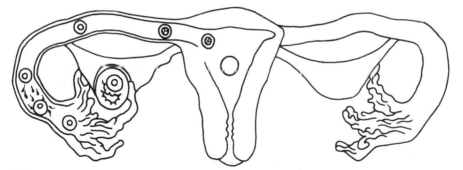

FIG. 5-1. Process of conception. The ovum is released from the ovary about 14 days prior to the menstrual period and begins its journey through the fallopian tube to the uterus. Propelled by their lashlike tails, the tiny sperm cells travel up through the cervix and uterus to where the ovum is located in the distal third of the fallopian tube. Fertilization can only occur if the sperm is less than 24 hours from ejaculation and the ovum has been released from the ovary within the previous 8 hours. Once conception occurs the cells immediately begin to differentiate and divide so that by the time the **conceptus** reaches the uterus it is ready to begin the process of implantation (Birth Atlas. New York, Maternity Center Association)

The new individual is already complete in that the two original cells from mother and father contain all the plans for how it will grow and develop into a baby. Hair, eyes, sex, blood type—all the inherited characteristics—are already determined. The embryo begins immediately to divide into various cells, becoming more and more dense instead of larger and larger so that it can continue its journey through the tube to the uterus and still be ready for implantation.

Have any of you ever heard of a tubal pregnancy? That is what happens when the mother has had some difficulty with the fallopian tube, such as an infection or surgery, which partially blocks it. Then the conceptus cannot pass through the tube and begins to grow there. Because the tube cannot expand the way the uterus can, the conceptus has to be removed by surgery.

After its journey through the tube, or about a week before the next period would normally occur, the embryo comes into the fundus and burrows its way into the lining of the uterus, which has been prepared for it. For a while, it lives on its own yolk sac, just like an unborn chick, but a communication system whereby the embryo can get nourishment from the mother's body is being prepared. The organ that is formed for this purpose is called the placenta, or afterbirth. It is a complex organ with a dull side, which grows into the uterine lining, and a shiny side, which is toward the baby. The spongelike placenta has a ropelike cord coming from its center to the baby's umbilicus, or belly button. The food and oxygen needed for the baby's growth and development are carried through the mother's bloodstream to the placenta, where they are filtered and carried to the baby through the umbilical cord. After the baby uses what it needs, its waste products travel back through the cord to the placenta. There they are once again filtered and carried away by the mother's bloodstream to be excreted through the mother's kidneys and, in the case of oxygen/carbon dioxide, through her lungs. You can easily see how this puts extra demands upon the mother while she is pregnant.

This filtering systems in the placenta protects the fetus. Although not as efficient as originally believed, the placental barrier does filter out bacteria and does not allow the baby's blood to mix directly with the mother's blood until the placenta begins to come away from the uterus at the time of delivery. This is important if the mother has a bacterial infection, or if she is Rh negative and the baby is Rh positive.

The shiny side of the placenta is a layer of membrane that extends to envelop the developing baby in a sac. This is called the amniotic sac, or the amnion, and contains a colorless fluid that is called amniotic fluid. Sometimes called the bag of waters, it keeps the baby in a safe, sterile, temperature-controlled environment. Since the fluid tension keeps the uterine walls from clinging tightly to the baby, there is room for growth and movement as well as protection from any outside blows.

Additional protection for the baby is provided by a plug of mucus that seals off the cervix, that long, narrow, lower part of the uterus that allowed the sperm to pass through on its journey toward the ovum, so that no bacteria or other infectious organisms can enter the uterus from the vagina. Because of this protection, intercourse up until term is allowed by many doctors in the absence of complications.

The tiny embryo is about the size of the head of a pin when the first period is missed, or about 1 week after implantation. At 6 weeks, the developing eye can be identified, as well as arm and leg buds and what will be the nose and mouth. The spine is prominent, the brain and nervous system being one of the earliest systems to be laid down. In fact, all the major systems are laid down in the first 3 months; after this time it is mainly a matter of growth and development of systems that are already formed. This is why the first 3 months are so crucial to the future infant.

If you look at an illustration of a fetus at about the third or fourth month, it appears to be a tiny, perfectly formed baby. By the fourth month, it is 8–10 inches long and weighs about 6 oz. The mother begins to feel her child move near the end of this time, and her body begins to show visible signs of pregnancy.

By the end of the sixth month, the **fundus** has reached as high as the mother's naval. The growing uterus has come up out of the pelvis, and the pressure against the bladder is relieved for a while. The baby has reached about a foot in length, and downy hair and fingernails have formed.

By the end of the seventh month, the baby could survive if it were born, but would need the specialized environment of a premature nursery. It has not yet laid down a layer of fat to insulate it and help keep the body temperature constant. Its facial and jaw muscles may not be strong enough to suck nourishment through a nipple, so it would need to be fed through a tube until the muscles developed more. Also, it does not yet have any resistance to infections.

This sample lecture is an example of how one teacher presented her material to a typical middle income group. How the baby grows and how it looks at the precise stage of pregnancy she is in is a source of endless fascination to the pregnant woman. She can be helped to fantasize, an important part of the middle trimester, if the instructor refers to the conceptus as "your baby" rather than "the fetus."

Nutrition

Eating Habits

To ensure that the mother is not nutritionally deficient in any significant way, the ideal time to assess her eating patterns would be several months prior to conception. However, although information about nutrition is widely available in books written for the general public, few couples pay any attention to their own nutrition until the baby is on the way. After any initial nausea has passed, the expectant mother is highly motivated to learn about a balanced diet.

The effects of nutritional excellance upon the health of the infant have been well established. Impressive evidence has also been presented that good nutrition helps make labor easier and lowers the rate of toxemia, prematurity, and stillbirth.[11,12] Many of the discomforts of pregnancy such as nausea, leg cramping, and fluid retention may often be prevented by an adequate diet or corrected by an improved diet.

Others in the health team will probably initiate nutrition counseling under the direction of the physician, but the childbirth educator is in a unique position to build up rapport with the expectant parents and can reinforce what other members of the maternal health team have begun. Too often the pregnant woman is merely given a printed sheet with dietary information. There may be little or no follow-up until or unless she runs into difficulty because of rapid weight gain or retention of fluids. Even then, the first recourse is usually to pharmacologic agents rather than dietary intervention. Although research into the effects of prenatal diet has been going on for nearly four decades, surprisingly little seems to have been practically implemented.

If this area has not been adequately covered by others on the maternal health team, it is worthwhile to devote at least part of a session to eating habits. Such a discussion may legitimately be placed into the "pregnancy as a state of health" framework.

Motivating to Improve Diet

The childbirth educator can learn a great deal about the parents' current eating patterns by having the mother bring in a record of everything she has eaten in a given 24-hour period. This record serves as a springboard for discussion and involves the expectant parents in planning their own diet around their individual food preferences.

Analysing current eating patterns, learning how to plan a balanced diet, and changing eating habits that have evolved since early childhood are bothersome tasks, and the pregnant woman will not willingly undertake them unless she realizes the importance of her nutritional status. This may be especially true for the woman who can ill afford high-quality protein foods and usually substitutes "filling" carbohydrates and coffee for a lift. Obviously it is this woman who is most likely to be nutritionally deficient to begin with and therefore most in need of a therapeutic diet. Unless it can be made clear to her that what she eats is of crucial importance to the future well-being of her infant as well as the course of her own pregnancy, she will not be likely to follow good advice about nutrition. She needs to know that she *can* affect the health of her child by eating a balanced diet and that by so doing she is doing her absolute best for her child. The task of the childbirth educator is one of motivating the expectant mother to learn, then to use what she has learned.

Balancing the Diet

Of crucial importance during pregnancy and lactation is the consumption of sufficient protein to meet the increased needs of the woman and the fetus. An intake of about 80 to 85 g of protein per day is recommended, and protein from each of the four basic food groups should be included. Even a cursory glance at protein equivalency charts shows that meeting this recommended amount takes planning. The woman who is reluctant to drink milk will find this especially difficult because a quart of milk supplies 32 to 35 g of protein. Although her calcium requirement can be met through calcium supplements, these supplements to not replace the protein lost if milk is deleted from her diet.

High-quality proteins, that is, those most complete in the amino acids needed to build tissue, are also the most expensive part of the diet. Fresh meats, poultry, or fish should be consumed daily. Other rich sources of protein are eggs and milk. Less protein is available from vegetable sources.

Incomplete protein sources, such as whole grains and legumes, have amino acid combinations that are not complete and so are not metabolized for body growth unless other sources supply the missing amino acids *simultaneously*. Ingestion of an incomplete protein at one meal and its complement at another meal is useless, because the body is incapable of retaining amino acids even if they are eaten within the same day. This makes it mandatory for the expectant mother who may wish to meet all or a large proportion of her protein needs from nonmeat sources to study carefully the complementary patterns before planning her diet. An excellent resource for this type of planning is *Diet for a Small Planet*, readily available in paperback in most bookstores.[7]

Efforts to limit weight gain frequently mean excessive emphasis on caloric control. The relationship between use of protein and adequate caloric intake should be kept in mind, however. If the expectant mother drastically limits her carbohydrates in an effort to maintain or even lose weight, proteins are diverted to fulfill her energy needs instead of being used for tissue growth. This reduces her available protein even further.

It is recommended that the pregnant woman have a minimum of 2000 calories per day. Of these, about 40% should come from high-quality proteins (meat, fish, poultry, milk, eggs), about 30% from fats or oils, and the remainder from the fruit, vegetable, cereal, and bread groups.

Because the numerous daily nutritional needs require quite a high caloric intake by themselves, few pregnant women can afford to indulge in nutritionally poor, highly refined sweets and starches. In order to get the most nourishment out of each calorie, the pregnant woman should eat the more natural foods, which usually have fewer chemical additives as well. For example, the caloric content of a 1-oz slice of white bread is similar to that of whole grain bread of the same weight. However, the natural B vitamins have been refined out of the white flour in processing, and the bread may have been enriched by the addition of artificial vitamins. The same is true of white rice *versus* brown rice, or white flour *versus* whole wheat flour for baking.

Sample Diet

The sample pregnancy diet (Table 5-1) gives a general outline of the foods that should be included every day. Since each person's nutritional status is different at the outset, additions or deletions to a pregnancy diet should be made by the nutritional counselor on an individual basis.

Table 5-1. **Sample Diet**

Food	Daily Amount	Comments
Milk	1 quart whole	The fat content in whole milk aids in the absorption of fat-soluble vitamins A and D from the milk. The woman who dislikes milk or who is lactose intolerant may substitute a 1-oz cube of hard cheese for 1 cup of her milk allowance per day. Dried milk powder equivalent to 1 quart liquid may be added to other foods. If skim milk should be prescribed, she should be aware that fat-free or skimmed milk has more protein than the popular skimmed milk products.
Eggs	1 or 2	Eggs are a relatively inexpensive source of high-quality protein.
Meats	6-8 oz	Lean meat, fish, or poultry, preferably in two servings. Liver once weekly is desirable. Baking or broiling retains vitamins best.
Fats	2 tbs	Unsaturated vegetable oils such as safflower or soya are preferred.
Vegetables	3-4 servings	At least one dark green or deep yellow vegetable should be eaten daily. To retain the most vitamins and minerals, brief steaming is most effective. Otherwise, baking or boiling in a minimum of water for the briefest possible time is best. Vegetable waters may be saved to conserve the nutrients lost into them and used later in soups or in cooking such foods as rice.
Fruits	2 servings	At least one citrus fruit should be eaten daily. Fresh fruits are preferred. If she uses canned products, the pregnant woman should read labels for sugar content and additives. Many companies now pack fruit in its own juice rather than heavy, sweet syrup, and the expectant mother can use these products to cut down on unnecessary sugar intake. Dried fruits such as prunes or apricots are relatively high in calories, but are excellent sources of iron.
Breads Cereals	3 servings	Whole grain products are preferred. The pregnant woman should read labels so that she can avoid unnecessary additives. The grains eaten should be varied among wheat, rye, corn, barley, oats, and rice.

(Modified from Your Pregnancy. Raritan, NJ, Ortho Pharmaceutical Corp, 1974)

In summary, the facts that the childbirth educator (who is not the primary nutrition counselor) should know are

1. The importance of monitoring for proper, expected weight control (the pregnant woman *should* gain at least 28 lb)
2. The need for adequate high-quality protein to meet the needs of mother and fetus
3. The need for an adequate caloric intake to metabolize the protein so that it can be used by the body

4. The need for a balanced and varied diet that includes items from all the basic four groups

The childbirth educator is urged to keep abreast of current nutritional research. We are constantly learning more about the nutrient requirements for healthy baby building as well as potential sources of danger in the form of pollutants, be they in the air or in the processing and preserving of the foods we eat. Some reading about nutrition that may be recommended for expectant parents is listed in Appendix C.

Physical Conditioning

Childbearing is a physical event similar in some respects to an athletic event requiring intense effort and stamina. The body is asked to perform under stress conditions over a period of hours. How well it is able to do so is determined in part by the mother's physical condition.

No time is too early to begin a program of physical conditioning. If physical exercise is not a part of the expectant mother's normal activity, limbering up exercises should be begun as early as possible to improve muscle tone, posture, circulation, and general mobility of joints. Such exercises also enhance her feeling of well-being and reinforce her attitude toward pregnancy as a healthy, normal state. The ideal of a continuum including pregnancy, childbearing, and the postnatal period can be applied here: physical preparation for the exertions of labor and delivery, physical performance during labor and delivery and physical recovery during involution.

Posture

The most frequent cause of backache in the pregnant woman is poor posture. When the body is in good alignment, a large proportion of the weight of the fundus rests in the pelvic basin, with the buttocks tucked under, the pelvis in a tilt position, and abdominal muscles supporting the fundus. The body weight is carried slightly anterior to the instep. The head is held erect and the shoulders well back to allow for adequate expansion of the rib cage (Fig. 5-2).

Frequently, however, as her increasing girth pulls her center of gravity toward the front, the woman reacts by relaxing her abdominal muscles, thereby increasing the already exaggerated curvature of the spine and shortening the muscles of her lower back (Fig. 5-3). She must then compensate by leaning backward slightly from the waist and by walking with her weight on her heels. This results in an ungainly waddling gait, as well as fatigue in the lower back.

To correct this difficulty, the pelvic tilt may be taught in a standing position. To acquire a feel for this maneuver, the student places one hand just below her back waist and the other underneath the fundus (or above the

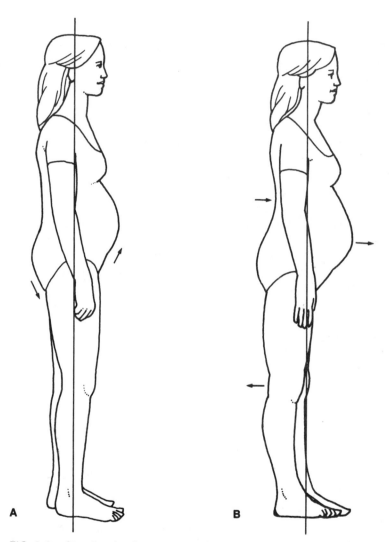

FIG. 5-2. Standing in alignment. (*A*) Good alignment. The pelvis is in a posterior tilt position, the abdominal muscles contracted, knees relaxed. The chin is tucked. The plumb line passes through the center of the body in good alignment. The weight is evenly distributed and carried at or slightly anterior to the arch of the foot. (*B*) Poor alignment. The abdominal muscles are relaxed, the knees locked back. The weight of the uterus falls forward, accentuating the common **lordotic** stance of late pregnancy. Because most of the weight is carried anterior to the center of gravity (represented by the plumb line), the tendency is to lean the upper body back and to walk with the weight posterior to the arch or on the heels.

symphysis if in early pregnancy). She begins by inhaling, then tilts the pelvis while exhaling by tucking in her buttocks and tilting her hips upward in front. If she does this by pulling up with the rectus abdominus, the resultant downward pull of the ribcage may cause some constriction of respiration. In this case she may be instructed to inhale deeply and practice the pelvic tilt while holding her breath for several seconds. She then learns to accomplish the tilt with less contraction of the rectus abdominus, relying instead on the external and internal obliques to tilt the anterior pelvis up.

Another teaching approach is to instruct the student to stand with her feet about 12 inches from the wall, leaning her back against the wall. She

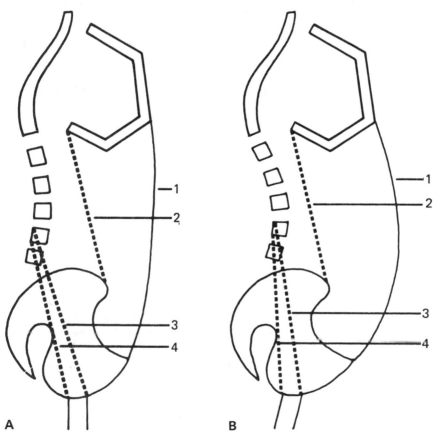

FIG. 5-3. (A)Good alignment. The rectus abdominus (1) and the external and internal oblique muscles (2) hold the pelvis in a posterior tilt position. The back and iliopsoas muscles (3) stretch passively. The rectus femoris (4) is relaxed, allowing the distal end of the femur to move anteriorly and causing the knee to relax. The curvature of the spine is minimized. (B) Poor alignment. The rectus abdominus (1) and the internal and external obliques (2) are relaxed, allowing the weight of the fundus to fall forward. The back and iliopsoas muscles (3) are shortened, pulling the pelvis forward. The rectus femoris (4) contracts, pulling the distal end of the femur posteriorly and allowing the knee to lock.

can then slide her hand down her back to find where the spine curves away from the wall. She then flattens her entire back against the wall while exhaling and holds this position. Placing her hands against the wall, she pushes away from it while maintaining the pelvic tilt position.

To bring the entire body into good alignment, the woman may be instructed to stand straight with her feet a few inches apart, her weight resting slightly anterior to her instep. While exhaling slowly, she rotates the head, bringing it forward, to the left, back, to the right side, then balancing it directly over the cervical spine with her eyes straight ahead. She can then rotate her arms and shoulders by bringing her arms straight out in front of her, then up over her head, back around as far as they will comfortably go, then dropping them to rest at her sides. This brings the shoulders into alignment. Following this, the pelvis should be brought into a tilt position if it is not already, and the knees relaxed. The woman should be encouraged to practice standing and walking in this position until it becomes natural.

To check for alignment, imagine a plumb line dropping from the top of the head, through the ear lobe, shoulder joint, hip socket just behind the patella, and anterior to the lateral malleolus (see Fig. 5-2).

Body Mechanics

Like good posture, body mechanics involve using the body properly to distribute stress evenly and to avoid overstressing any one muscle group. If she follows the principle of keeping the body in a balanced position with the weight evenly distributed, the pregnant woman can use her body most efficiently while pursuing the various activities of her daily life. It is preferable for the woman to squat rather than stoop if she desires to pick up something from the floor. Besides putting her off balance, a stooping posture requires the back muscles to pull the weight of the trunk upward. The leg muscles do the work of pushing her back into a standing position from a squat (Fig. 5-4). Similarly, if a work surface is too low (*e.g.*, while making a bed), she should bend at the knees rather than at the waist.

Lifting. When lifting a heavy object, the pregnant woman should always bring it in close to her body to avoid stressing the lower back muscles. Bringing it as close as possible to the center of gravity distributes the weight evenly. For example, to lift a toddler, the woman should first squat down to his or her level, draw the child close to her body, then let her legs push her up. The same procedure applies if the object is somewhat higher, like a chair. The knees should be bent until the trunk is at the same level as the object; then, keeping the spine straight, the object is pulled in close to the body and the knees straightened. When lifting or carrying unwieldy objects such as groceries, care should be taken to see that they are evenly distributed. Two lighter bags are preferable to one heavy one.

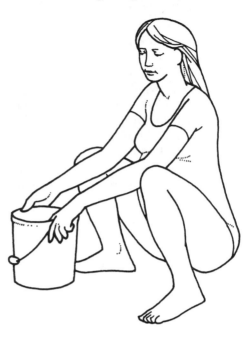

FIG. 5–4. Squatting. When reaching for a low object, the pregnant woman should squat, keeping her back straight and her body in good alignment. The object should then be pulled in close to her body. When she stands up again, the legs do the work of propelling her upward.

Climbing Stairs.   To maintain good body alignment while climbing stairs, the weight is first transferred to the forward foot, then the knee is straightened fully while the lower knee is bent and brought forward in preparation for the next step. The pelvis is kept in a tilt position with the spine straight. This assures proper balance and forces the leg and foot muscles to do the work of propelling the body upward.

Rising.   To rise from a supine position, the woman may either roll onto her side and push herself into a sitting position with her hands or clasp her hands around her ankle with the knee bent and extend the leg slowly to pull herself into a sitting position. Neither of these methods puts strain on the back and abdominal muscles. From the sitting position, she progresses to a squat, then pushes up with her legs.

Rest and Relaxation

As pregnancy places increasing demands upon the woman's body, it is important for her to have adequate rest. She need not take long naps, but instead can allow herself several short rest periods during the day. Although many people feel that they cannot rest unless conditions are ideal, it is a skill that can be learned with a little practice.

Comfort Positions.   First, the woman must be in a comfortable position. She may assume any position in which all parts of her body are supported, that is no body part is resting on any other body part, and circulation is not interfered with in any way (Fig. 5-5). She can be **tailor sitting,** in a supine position well supported by pillows under shoulders and knees, or on her side with the pelvis tilted, both knees bent slightly, the upper one forward and resting on a pillow (this prevents overextension of the hip muscles). The weight of the fundus rests on the bed or mat. The head should be supported by a pillow, which may be angled to support the upper arm also. Other comfort positions include sitting in an armchair with feet and knees supported, head resting back, arms resting loosely at the sides, or even sitting at a desk with head leaning forward on the desk or a small pillow, arms crossed over the head, legs and feet relaxed.

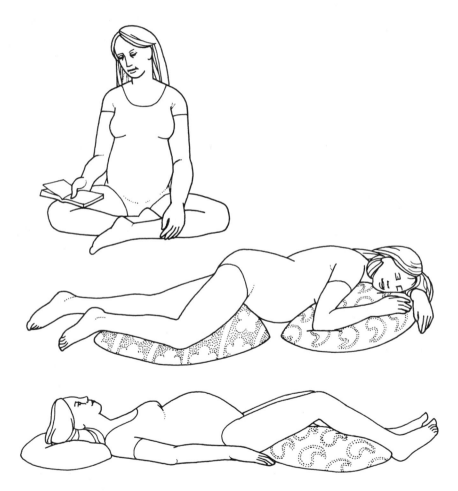

FIG. 5-5. Comfort positions. The comfort positions for pregnancy are positions in which the body is in alignment, with no body part resting on any other body part to interfere with circulation.

Achieving Relaxation. Once the comfort position is assumed, the woman should take a deep breath as a signal for relaxation, then consciously relax all of her voluntary muscles while she gently exhales. She can say to herself, "breathe out and relaaaax" as she does so.

While she is first learning to relax, she may need to check each muscle group and consciously let go of tension. If she is unsure that a muscle group is relaxed, she can contract it slightly, then release it and notice the difference. She might begin by checking feet, then, in turn, legs, thighs, buttocks, abdominal muscles, back, shoulders, arms, hands, neck, and end by making a face and relaxing again on a final exhalation. Following this, she must empty her mind of worry. This too takes some practice, but may be accomplished by concentrating on some peaceful scene (like a woodland pool), or on the quiet, effortless rhythm of her own breathing. By practicing diligently in exactly the same way each time and using the word *relax* on the exhalation, she eventually conditions herself to respond to the signal breath alone, which facilitates relaxation.

Problems Affecting Pregnancy Outcome

The old-fashioned approach to the possibility of complications in a pregnancy was to tell the mother as little as possible in order to prevent anxiety. It was assumed that the less she knew, the less she would worry. This "leave everything to the doctor" school of thought reduced the mother's psychological status to that of a child and gave the medical establishment the role of parent. Fortunately this attitude is waning.

Parents today are better informed, insisting upon explanation and demanding change when they feel it is justified. This is especially true of middle-class parents. Although information is available and free to anyone who can make use of a public library, radio, or television, the poor are less likely to see themselves as able to effect change.

If the mother is to share the responsibility for her health under the supervision of her doctor or clinic, she must be kept informed about possible problems so that complications may be reported promptly or avoided whenever possible. She also needs to be alerted to the dangers in the various pollutants, drugs, food additives, and so forth to which she may be exposed.

Some possible complications may be brought up as a result of questions from the class, which makes it easy for the instructor. In less vocal classes or in classes where the parents do not really see themselves as participants in the learning process, the instructor must initiate discussion. The fact that the class does not volunteer questions about complications by no means indicates that this topic is not one of concern to them. Every pregnant woman wonders if her baby will be healthy. Primigravidas may wonder if they are capable of producing a perfect baby; multigravidas may wonder if they can do it again. This is a sensitive area and one in which the instructor may well have to detect the unasked question. Reassurance comes with knowledge.

Early or middle pregnancy classes are primarily concerned with problems that affect the outcome of the pregnancy. Many tragic birth defects are the result of disturbances in the prenatal environment, some of which could have been avoided if the mother had been aware of the danger.

Chemical Agents

A case in point is the ingestion of **teratogens.** Any chemical that is dissolved in the mother's bloodstream readily crosses the placenta and enters the baby's bloodstream. Such chemicals include prescription and nonprescription drugs, food additives and pollutants, alcohol, and nicotine derived from smoking (Table 5-2).

Drugs. The world is well aware of the tragic effects of thalidomide. It is far less aware of the noxious effects of insecticides that the expectant mother may spray around her kitchen or picnic site. Not every child born of a mother who has been exposed to noxious chemicals will be afflicted, however. Apgar found that some children appear to be uniquely susceptible owing to genetic predisposing factors.[2]

The greatest danger to the developing fetus from the teratogens is during the first trimester when the major systems are forming. The fact that the mother may be unaware of the pregnancy in these important early weeks is an excellent argument for planned parenthood.

Finding the cause of birth defects is rarely a simple procedure, partly because it is impossible to perform controlled laboratory studies on humans. Although animal studies give some indication of possible problems, laboratory studies on rats exonerated thalidomide as a source of abnormality for rat fetuses, so it is obvious that the results of tests on laboratory animals do not always apply to humans. Additionally, even drugs that have been demonstrated to be damaging may cause problems in only a small percentage of those exposed to it. Until a drug has been *proven* innocent, it is wise to forgo all medications except those specifically prescribed by a physican who is aware of the pregnancy. This includes such household staples as aspirin, which has been implicated in newborn clotting difficulties when the mother has taken it near term. Also, over-the-counter remedies should be avoided; even Neo-Synephrine nasal spray, when used repeatedly, has been known to raise a pregnant woman's blood pressure.

The fact that chemicals cross the placenta readily is beneficial in some instances because the fetus can be treated at the same time as the mother. A good example is the penicillin treatment of the syphilitic mother.

Table 5-2. **Drugs Adversely Affecting the Human Fetus**

Drugs	Adverse effects	Comments
Analgesics		
Heroin and morphine	When taken near term: respiratory depression, neonatal death, addiction	Fairly well documented
Salicylates	When taken near term: neonatal bleeding, coagulation defects	
Anesthetics		
Mepivacaine	When taken near term: fetal bradycardia, neonatal respiratory depression	More studies needed
Antibacterials		
Chloramphenicol	When taken near term: gray syndrome, death	Fairly well documented
Nitrofurantoin	When taken near term: hemolysis	More studies needed
Novobiocin	When taken near term; hyperbilirubinemia	More studies needed
Streptomycin	Throughout pregnancy: 8th nerve damage, hearing loss, multiple skeletal anomalies	Debatable, more studies needed
Sulfonamides (long acting)	When taken near term: hyperbilirubinemia, kernicterus	Fairly well documented
Tetracyclines	When taken in 2nd and 3rd trimesters: inhibition of bone growth, discoloration of teeth	Fairly well documented
Anticarcinogens		
Amethopterin	When taken in 1st trimester: cleft palate, abortion	Fairly well documented
Aminopterin	When taken in 1st trimester: cleft palate, abortion	Known teratogen
Cyclophosphamide	When taken in 1st trimester: severe stunting, fetal death, extremity defects	More studies needed
Anticoagulants		
Warfarin	Throughout pregnancy: fetal death, hemorrhage	More studies needed
Antidiabetics		
Chlorpropamide	Throughout pregnancy: prolonged neonatal hypoglycemia	More evidence needed
Tolbutamide	Throughout pregnancy: congenital anomalies	One reported case only; evidence lacking

(continued)

Table 5-2. **Drugs Adversely Affecting the Human Fetus** *(continued)*

Drugs	Adverse effects	Comments
Antimalarials		
Quinine	Deafness	More studies needed
Antimitotic Agents		
Podophyllum	Fetal resorption, multiple deformities	More studies needed
Antithyroid Agents		
Methimazole	When taken from 14th week on: goiter and mental retardation	Fairly well documented
Potassium iodide	When taken from 14th week on: goiter and mental retardation	Fairly well documented
Propylthiouracil	When taken from 14th week on: goiter and mental retardation	Fairly well documented
Radioactive iodine	When taken from 14th week on: congenital hypothyroidism	Fairly well documented
Depressants		
Phenobarbital	When taken in excessive amounts: neonatal bleeding, increased rate of neonatal drug metabolism	
Reserpine	When taken near term: nasal block	One report only, more studies needed
Thalidomide	When taken 28th–42nd day: phocomelia, hearing defects	Known teratogen
Diuretics		
Ammonium chloride	Acidosis	
Thiazides (hydrochlorothiazide, chlorothiazide, methyclothiazide)	In latter part of pregnancy: thrombocytopenia, neonatal death	One report only, evidence lacking
Stimulants		
Dextroamphetamine sulfate	Transposition of great vessels	One report only
Phenmetrazine	When taken 4th–12th week: skeletal and visceral anomalies	One report only
Sex steroids		
Androgens, estrogens, and oral progestogens	Masculinization and labial fusion (early in pregnancy), clitoris enlargement (later in pregnancy)	Fairly well documented

(continued)

Table 5–2. **Drugs Adversely Affecting the Human Fetus** *(continued)*

Drugs	Adverse effects	Comments
Miscellaneous		
Acetophenetidin	Methemoglobinemia	More studies needed
Cholinesterase inhibitors	Throughout pregnancy: transient muscular weakness	More studies needed
Hexamethonium bromide	Throughout pregnancy: neonatal ileus, death	More studies needed
Iophenoxic acid	Elevated serum protein-bound iodine	
Isonicotinic acid hydrazide (INH)	Retarded psychomotor activity	More studies needed
Lysergic acid diethylamide (LSD)	When taken in 1st trimester: chromosomal damage, stunted offspring	More studies needed
Nicotine and smoking	Throughout pregnancy: low-birth-weight babies	More studies needed
Vitamin A	Throughout pregnancy: congenital anomalies, cleft palate, eye damage, syndactyly	In large doses only
Vitamin D	Throughout pregnancy: excessive blood calcium, mental retardation	In large doses only
Vitamin K analogues	When taken near term: hyperbilirubinemia, kernicterus	In large doses

(Adapted from Drugs Adversely Affecting the Human Fetus (abstr). Columbus, Ross Laboratories, 1971. *Original sources:* Mirkin B: Postgrad Med 47:91, 1970; Takata A: Hosp Formulary Mgt 4:25, 1969)

Food Additives. Food additives such as cyclamate and monosodium glutamate have been shown to cause abnormalities in animal studies. Admittedly, abnormalities have only been demonstrated when these additives were administered in huge doses, but who is to judge how much is too much for an individual fetus? No mother would willingly risk the future health of her unborn baby is she were aware of the danger.

Pregnancy often motivates a woman to read labels on packaged and processed foods. Many additives that have not been proven innocent are likely to appear; the only purpose of many of these, such as carrageenan in frozen dairy products, is to lengthen the self life of an item in the store. Others, such as the bright orange dye used in orange soda, are added solely for eye appeal.

If the expectant mother begins to read labels during her pregnancy, she becomes aware of other additives that, although not harmful, she may not particularly want as a part of every food she and her family eat. For example, many baby foods still contain salt and monosodium glutamate as a part of their usual makeup. The mother may not feel that these make a valuable addition to the baby's diet, and reading labels helps her to avoid them. Sugar is also included in unexpected places. A reading of cereal labels reveals that almost every cold cereal, with the exception of shredded wheat, includes sugar as an important ingredient.

Narcotics. Although heroin has not been shown to cause birth defects other than those associated with poor nutrition, the infant born to the addicted mother must suffer withdrawal symptoms after birth. The same holds true for the infant whose mother is on methadone. These infants are usually of low birth weight and must be treated as addicts, usually by withdrawing them gradually with decreasing doses of paregoric or, in less grave cases, of phenobarbital. The infant whose mother has been withdrawn immediately prior to his birth may be in even greater danger unless his needs are immediately recognized and he is himself withdrawn as a separate entity.

The physician who is overseeing the woman's prenatal care has the primary responsibility for recognizing these cases. However, health care is sometimes fragmented, especially when the expectant mother is attending a public facility rather than establishing a rapport with one physician or midwife. If the childbirth educator becomes aware that the parturient is on illicit drugs and suspects that the attending physician is not informed, she should strongly encourage the woman to tell her physician for the sake of the infant.

Smoking. Although smoking cigarettes has long been recognized as deleterious to both the expectant mother and to the baby, very little responsibility has been taken by the medical community to encourage pregnant women to give it up. Simply telling a woman to stop is ineffective because it neither enlists her active participation nor demonstrates continued interest on the part of the health care giver. Acquainting her with the alarming results of studies done on infants of mothers who smoked during pregnancy will give her motivation to improve her fetus' prenatal environment, if she will not stop for her own sake.

Hesitation on our part for fear of alarming the expectant mother should be outweighed by the positive health effects if she stops smoking or cuts down her consumption.

Cigarette smoke contains more than 1000 drugs, including cyanide and carbon monoxide—drugs to which nobody would willingly expose themselves or their children. The effects of smoking cigarettes (or exposure to cigarette smoke) include fetal growth retardation and increased risk of fetal or neonatal death as well as a number of adaptational problems in the neonatal period. Results of recent research, both here and abroad, indicate that fetal deaths linked to maternal smoking are most frequently attributed to "unknown" causes or to anoxia, while the perinatal deaths are caused by premature delivery or respiratory difficulty. Furthermore, studies have shown strong associations between sudden infant death syndrome (SIDS) and the frequency and level of maternal smoking during pregnancy. One study suggested linkage between maternal smoking in the postpartum period and SIDS.[10]

Children of mothers who smoked during pregnancy have been found to have significantly lower IQ scores and an increased incidence of reading disorders, minimal brain dysfunction (MBD), and hyperkinesis than offspring of nonsmokers, even when matched for age, parity, and socioeconomic factors. These results suggest that fetal central nervous system development may be impaired owing to maternal smoking.[1]

The undesirable effects of smoking on the mother are generally well known, including increased risk of bronchitis, emphysemia, lung cancer, cardiopulmonary and cardiovascular disease, arteriosclerosis, bladder cancers, and peptic ulcers. During pregnancy, in addition, smoking markedly increases the risk of serious complications. Even prior to conception, it was found, women who smoked had an increased risk of abnormal implantation (placenta previa) and of large areas of dead tissue on the placenta.[9] Abruptio placentae (with its 10% mortality rate) is found to increase by 24% in moderate smokers and by 68% in heavy smokers.

The two drugs contained in cigarette smoke that apparently cause the most damage are nicotine and carbon monoxide. Cigarette smoking causes rises in plasma arterial nicotine, which in turn causes vasoconstriction of the microcirculation, including the uterine vascular bed.[10] Studies done on pregnant primates show that nicotine causes a profound reduction in uterine blood flow and a corresponding fall in fetal Po_2. Interestingly, the Po_2 does not alter significantly in the maternal bloodstream, but shows a 25% greater decrease in the fetus. Tobacco smoke exposure, like nicotine injection, reduces fetal breathing movements, a result of the fall in fetal Po_2. Thermographic studies likewise show an apparent decrease in placental blood flow during smoking.

Carbon monoxide acts by binding the O_2-carrying hemoglobin with a far greater affinity than O_2, forming the stable compound carboxyhemoglobin, thus reducing the O_2-carrying capacity of the blood. In addition, carbon monoxide diffuses across the placenta and combines with fetal hemoglobin, reducing fetal O_2-carrying capacity even further. Because of the pressure gradient of placental exchange, carboxyhemoglobin levels are higher in the fetus than in the mother.

It seems likely that the reduced O_2 available to the fetus because of the effects of nicotine (vasoconstriction of placental bed) is added to the reduced carrying capacity of maternal and fetal hemoglobin due to carbon monoxide to cause the adverse effects on fetal development.

As childbirth educators we owe it to our clients to present the serious nature of the risks resulting from cigarette smoking to mother and infant. Ideally, this begins as soon as the expectant mother comes for prenatal care, with recognition of the smoker, and education and support for her efforts to stop. Note that passive inhalation of the smoke exhaled by others likewise has been shown to result in significant rises in both maternal nicotine and carboxyhemoglobin levels.

As health care providers, we need to demonstrate our commitment to the adverse effects of smoking by not smoking ourselves and by not allowing smoking in areas (such as in waiting rooms) where pregnant women may be exposed to tobacco smoke. In our own communities, we should find out if smoke cessation groups or clinics exist so they may be used for referral. Finally, continuing interest and support for the smoker who is trying to stop may be essential for her success.

Alcohol. When taken in moderate amounts, alcohol has not been proven to have major undesirable effects upon the fetus. However, we really do not know if there is a safe lower limit of consumption. Although we generally think of the woman who is a chronic alcoholic as the one who is likely to produce an infant with fetal alcohol syndrome, it seems that the woman who customarily drinks 1 to 3 oz of alcohol per day has a 10% to 20% chance of producing an infant with characteristics of fetal alcohol syndrome (growth deficiency, facial and joint malformations, significantly lower IQ), and reports have been made of an occasional woman who habitually abstained from alcohol but who indulged in binging during her pregnancy and delivered a child with fetal alcohol syndrome. It seems likely that elements of dosage, timing, and a vulnerable fetus combine to determine which child will be afflicted.

Although we do not have enough hard evidence to forbid consumption of alcohol entirely, the wise course would seem to be to limit consumption to no more than an occasional glass of wine or beer.

Infectious Diseases

Most illnesses that are contracted by the mother are responded to by her own immunologic system and are not injurious to the fetus. A few, such as rubella, cytomegalovirus, and toxoplasmosis, do attack the fetus with grave results.

Rubella. As in the case of the teratogens, the amount and kind of damage rubella inflicts on the fetus varies according to the developmental phase of the fetus at the time of exposure and possibly any congenital predisposition that renders a particular fetus vulnerable. Not every unborn baby exposed to rubella will be born with a defect. One study made on 19 families with a child who was deaf as a result of prenatal exposure to rubella showed that in 13 of the 19 families at least one parent had hereditary hearing abnormalities and in only 5 of the families were there no hereditary traits associated with deafness.[2]

Except for the first trimester, where the incidence of malformation after exposure to rubella is about 50%, the chances that the infant will be defective decrease with each prenatal month. Many physicians now do routine screening for rubella titers (available free from the Board of Health) as a part of their prenatal workup early in pregnancy to find out whether the mother has had rubella in the past. Later testing can rule out rubella if infections occur during the gestational period. If it can be demonstrated that the mother has the infection during the first trimester of her pregnancy, a termination of the pregnancy may be considered.

Toxoplasmosis.   Toxoplasmosis is another infectious disease that has been indicted in birth defects. This disease, little noted by adults who contract it, may cause a rash, lymphadenopathy, or upper respiratory symptoms for a few days. It has disastrous consequences for the fetus, however. "Of the unborn infants who do have toxoplasmosis during pregnancy, about 20% are born with major defects including mental retardation, hydrocephalus, epilepsy, eye damage, and hearing loss."[2]

Toxoplasmosis may be prevented by scrupulously avoiding sources of infection such as raw meat. Since the causative organisms are killed by heat over 140 degrees, the expectant mother should always eat her meat well done if she is eating out or cooked to the 140 degree mark on a meat thermometer if she is cooking at home.

Another source of this infection is the feces of cats. If the couple owns a cat, the expectant mother should not be the one to clean out the liter box. The cat can be tested by a veterinarian for toxoplasmosis, but since it can be infected at any time through contact with other cats or eating rare meat (or mice), it seems sensible for the mother to avoid all contact with cat feces. Digging in a garden that may have been contaminated by neighborhood cats and contact with strange cats may also be avoided as precautionary measures.

Prevention of Infectious Diseases.   There are other infectious diseases, such as cytomegalic inclusion disease, which can cause serious damage to the unborn child, even death or miscarriage. Unfortunately, there are fewer decisive measures to prevent them. Seeing that every woman contracts or is immunized against rubella, measles, whooping cough, mumps, poliomyelitis, diphtheria, and smallpox prior to any possible pregnancy is the surest prevention. Pregnancy should be avoided for 3 months following rubella immunization. Information about infectious diseases should be included in any discussion of family planning.

Toxemia

Toxemia is a disease of unknown etiology that occurs in pregnancy and the puerperium. It is characterized by rapid weight gain and mild **edema** in the early phases, due to sodium retention. This is followed by a generalized **vasoconstriction** plus increased sodium retention and a decrease in plasma volume. If unchecked, it can progress to the graver symptoms of vasoconstriction: convulsions or coma resulting from cerebral ischemia, a decrease in urinary output resulting from vasoconstriction of renal circulation, and interference with maternal–fetal circulation.

Traditional therapy included sodium restriction and the use of **diuretics.** Recent studies demonstrating the possible side-effects of the diuretics have led physcans to discontinue using them, however. In addition, there has been a great deal of controversy recently about the restriction of sodium. It is now felt that drastic sodium restriction is deleterious to the woman suffering from the concomitant hypovolemia found in the more advanced phase of the disease.

Currently, toxemia is treated with bed rest in the hope of increasing flow to the placental bed. Antihypertensive drugs are prescribed by some, although this is fairly controversial. The only true cure is delivery, if the fetus is sufficiently mature.

Although the cause of toxemia is still unproven, some researchers attribute it to nutritional deficiency.[12] It is established that this disease occurs more frequently in the poor, the malnourished, and those at the extremes in age. (One might conclude that the teen-age mother, with her own increased nutritional need, is competing with the fetus for nourishment.) Strangely, the one group with a lower toxemia rate is the heavy smokers. No explanation of this peculiarity has been offered.

Discussing the Physiologic Changes of Late Pregnancy

In keeping with our focus on current concerns, always begin with the immediate interest in order to validate that concern before moving on to other topics. The logical place to commence, if your class consists of expectant parents in the final trimester of pregnancy, will be with late pregnancy: how it feels to be near term (or have a wife who is nearing term) and what some of the underlying causes are of these feelings and discomforts.

Discussion techniques are useful for giving and gathering information at this point. Just about every symptom of late pregnancy mentioned in class will bring nods of agreement from some members of the group. This establishes common ground and increases class involvement. If these body changes can be discussed as the way the body is preparing for the work of labor and delivery, it is reassuring as well.

Respiratory Changes

As pregnancy progresses, the height of the fundus exerts indirect pressure against the diaphragm so that it is elevated from its normal position. This elevation causes a decrease in the space occupied by the lungs at the end of a normal expiration (the functional residual capacity). Concurrently, the thoracic cage expands outwardly, probably because of a greater mobility of the rib attachments, allowing for an increase in the tidal volume of air in each breath. This fact, along with the increased respiratory rate in the pregnant woman, results in a markedly increased minute volume, (*i.e.*, the *amount* of air exchanged in a minute).

One would expect that the increased demands of pregnancy would account for this, but in actual fact the increase in minute volume is larger than is necessary for the increased oxygen needs of the fetus, whereas the partial pressure of CO_2 is lower than in the nonpregnant state. Hellman and Pritchard suggest that this is probably due to the increased progesterone produced by the placenta, which has been shown to lower blood levels of CO_2, perhaps by acting upon the sensitivity of the respiratory center to CO_2 stimulation.[6] This normal hyperventilation found in pregnancy must be considered when teaching respiratory techniques for labor. Care must be taken not to compromise the respiratory exchange further by initiating a rate so rapid that it causes symptoms or by involving prolonged active expiration.

Symptoms of breathlessness are common in the third trimester. Some of this is attributable to the exertion of carrying around the 24 pounds or so the mother will have gained with the pregnancy, and some, to the increase in basal metabolism. Occasionally it may be due to constricting clothing, especially if the mother has not availed herself of a maternity brassiere commensurate with her increasing size. The mother may be advised to elevate the upper trunk so that the abdominal contents are not causing further pressure on the diaphragm.

Circulatory

By the third trimester, the weight of the **gravid** uterus is exerting considerable pressure on the pelvic veins and the inferior vena cava. This results in stagnation of blood in the lower extremities with increased venous pressure below the level of the inferior vena cava. The mild dependent edema of the legs and feet commonly seen at the end of the day in the last trimester is a direct effect of this. After a night's rest in the recumbent position, the edema has characteristically disappeared.

A more malignant effect is the development of varicosities in the legs or vulva. Contributing factors to this condition are the increased pressure caused by the pelvic contents and the **hypervolemia** of pregnancy; poor muscle tone, especially in the legs, because return circulation is assisted by the massaging action of the leg muscles; hereditary predisposition; and constricting clothing (slacks or garters, perhaps a panty girdle that has legs).

Even if the mother does not have varicosities, light support hose will increase her comfort in the final months. These may be bought in any hosiery store and are neither unsightly nor very expensive. The light massaging action of the elastic fiber in the hosiery helps to reduce fatigue and dependent edema of the feet. If she does have varicosities, she should be strongly encouraged to invest in true support hose, the kind available from pharmaceutical companies. It should be made clear to her that the benefits of preventing further damage, which may not recede after the birth, far outweigh the inconvenience of having to wear support hose for the limited duration of the pregnancy.

Postural measures for prevention or improvement of circulatory impairment include frequent elevation of the legs and feet. The mother can elevate her feet during several short rest periods during the day. If she has the opportunity, she might try resting on the floor or bed with her feet supported against the wall. A pillow under her hips helps, if this does not cause **dyspnea** by displacing the abdominal contents upward (Fig. 5-6).

If the mother has vulval varicosities, raising the hips is an important aid to postural venous drainage. In addition to using the pillow to raise her hips, she should raise her entire trunk for short periods to displace the weight of the uterus upward. If she has serious vulval varicosities, her physician will undoubtedly suggest a maternity girdle for good support because rupture of these varicose veins can cause major problems at delivery.

Especially if she has a problem with circulation from the lower extremities, the expectant mother should sleep on her side. The supine position does not relieve the vena cava and pelvic veins of the weight of the uterus (see Fig. 5-5).

Because of the delayed circulation, the woman may find that she feels dizzy if she gets up suddenly. She should rise slowly, using good body mechanics to allow time for homeostasis to occur.

Gastrointestinal Changes

As the uterus enlarges, the viscera are displaced from their usual positions by intra-abdominal pressure. In addition, progesterone being

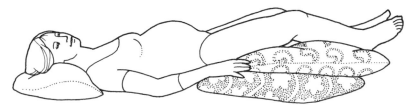

FIG. 5-6. For varicosities of the legs, legs should be elevated to enhance venous return. If vulval varicosities are present, the hips should be elevated as well.

produced by the placenta causes "generalized relaxation of smooth muscle, showing its effect in the gastrointestinal tract as well as in the uterus, ureters, and blood vessels."[6] These two factors contribute to a slowing down of gastrointestinal motility, or movement of the stomach contents into the intestines and peristaltic action in the intestine. The two most common complaints directly attributable to these conditions are heartburn and constipation.

Heartburn is probably due mainly to the displacement of the stomach as well as the delayed emptying time and is a result of regurgitation of acid stomach contents into the lower esophagus. Symptomatic relief in the form of an antacid may be prescribed by the physician. The expectant mother should be cautioned against taking bicarbonate of soda, which may be her customary measure for this complaint, because the high sodium content may cause fluid retention. The importance of good posture to avoid additional pressure on the stomach and allow it to function as efficiently as possible should also be explained.

Constipation is caused by decreased gastric motility, pelvic congestion due to impaired venous function, and perhaps to poor muscle tone. It should be treated promptly when it occurs. Another contributing factor is the addition of iron to the mother's daily vitamin supplement to meet her increased need for iron in the final trimester. The iron supplement is sometimes combined with a stool softener, which can help prevent constipation.

The mother should be encouraged to include enough fluid in her daily diet (about 6–8 glasses, one glass of water upon arising in the morning). She should also be sure to get enough roughage (whole grain cereals or breads) to give bulk to the stool. Prunes or licorice may help because of their mild laxative effect; some people experience a mild **catharsis** from spinach as well. The mother should be cautioned against the use of mineral oil as a laxative because it interferes with the absorption of lipid-soluble vitamins from the gastrointestinal tract.

Because sluggish venous circulation to the bowel contributes to constipation, Wiedenbach suggests that in addition to maintaining good body alignment, the expectant mother be instructed to contract the lower abdominal muscles in an inward and upward direction several times a day to improve venous flow.[14]

Increased estrogens during pregnancy are thought to be the cause of the increased vascularity and softening that are commonly seen in the gums. Often the gums are so friable that even a slight brush with a toothbrush can cause bleeding. Gingivitis is not uncommon, especially in the later months, and should be seen by a dentist, who may elect to cauterize the affected area.

If dental caries are present, the expectant mother may experience increased pain due to **hyperemia** of the gums, caused by her increased blood volume during pregnancy. This is not an effect of decalcification (old wives' tales to the contrary), which does not occur in fully calcified mature teeth.

Urinary Changes

In the first trimester, urinary frequency is caused by the pressure of the enlarging uterus on the bladder. As the fundus comes up out of the pelvis, this symptom lessens until **lightening** takes place. Then the bladder is squeezed between the heavy uterus and the **symphysis pubis,** and urinary frequency reappears.

There is no treatment. Some physicians recommend that the pregnant woman limit evening fluids if her sleep is disturbed by frequent urination. However, the fluid accumulated in the lower extremities during the day as dependent edema is usually reabsorbed at night, when the woman is recumbent. Since this reabsorbed fluid must also be excreted by the kidneys, limiting fluid intake is not too effective.

The mother is more susceptible to urinary tract infections during late pregnancy because pelvic pressure interferes with efficient circulatory and lymphatic drainage from the bladder. The pressure of the uterus sometimes causes a blockage of the ureter, especially on the right side. The urinary **stasis** may allow an increase in colon bacilli, normally present in the urinary tract, which occasionally leads to pyelonephritis.

Skin and Integumentary Changes

Many questions center around "stretch marks," the **striae gravidarum.** Reddish, slightly indented streaks, they appear primarily on the abdomen, but not infrequently on the breasts also. In the **multipara** the silvery scars of striae from previous pregnancies can also be seen. They are caused by rupture and retraction of the elastic fibers in the reticular portion of the dermis, well below the outer layers of the epidermis.

Little can be done to prevent these stretch marks from forming; some women seem to exhibit a predisposition and will develop more with subsequent pregnancies. The number of striae seems to correlate with the amount of enlargement that has taken place. Rubbing the skin with cocoa butter or other emollient helps to prevent the itching on the overstretched skin, but has no effect upon the formation of striae. The woman needs to be reassured that the striae lose their angry reddish appearance after birth, however.

Changes in pigmentation may be noted, influenced by **estrogen, progesterone,** and melanocyte-stimulating hormone from the pituitary. The dark area around the nipple becomes larger and darker, the **linea nigra** appears as a vertical streak on the abdomen from pubis to **umbilicus,** and brownish patches may appear on the face as a mask of pregnancy (**chloasma**). Some black women report that they actually become darker when they are pregnant. All of these pigmentary changes normalize after delivery, although some traces may remain if the changes were marked.

Although many women experience an improvement or no change in their complexions during pregnancy, the high estrogen levels trigger skin blemishes in others.

Vascular changes that show up in the skin include vascular spiders and **erythema** of the palms and soles of the feet. These may be accounted for by the combination of increased estrogen and intravascular pressure. These changes, too, recede after delivery.

Musculoskeletal Changes

Postural errors that result from the woman's changing center of gravity may lead to lordosis and mild backache (see Posture). By the third trimester, if uncorrected, these postural errors cause more marked symptoms and may, in addition, cause the woman to stand with her head forward and shoulders rounded. This anterior flexion of the neck, combined with slouching of the shoulder girdle, causes traction on the median and ulnar nerves, which results in a numbness or tingling sensation in the arms and hands.[3] The alignment exercises are helpful in this situation, with more attention to the upper trunk, head, and neck. Head and shoulder rotations are also useful.

Leg cramps are a common complaint in late pregnancy. Contributing factors include impaired circulation and inadequate calcium. The calcium deficiency may be due to poor calcium intake, to malabsorption, or to increased excretion of calcium due to an imbalance of the calcium-phosphorous ratio. When the phosphorous level is far in excess of the calcium level, the body rids itself of the excess phosphorous by combining it with calcium and excreting it in the urine. This further depletes the available calcium. Many of our most reliable sources of calcium, such as milk, supply even more phosphorous. Therefore, increasing the mother's milk intake simply adds to the problem. Her physician might have her limit her milk intake and supplement her diet with calcium tablets, or he may choose to order a medication, such as an aluminum hydroxide gel, to help her absorb some of the phosphorous. Leg cramps can also be produced by parathyroid deficiency or hyperventilation.

When cramping occurs, it may be treated instantly by flexing the ankle and forcing the toes upward. The knee must be straightened. If the woman is awakened by the cramp, as so frequently happens, she can find relief and go back to sleep if she straightens her leg and places her foot against a hard surface (e.g., the wall, or a head or foot board) so that it is held in flexion. Although a firm surface is preferable, a rolled pillow will do if a firm surface is unavailable.

Sometimes, cartilaginous relaxation permits mobility of the sacrococcygeal, pubic, or sacroiliac joints. Symptoms include pain over the joints and, in more severe cases, pain on walking and turning over in bed. Relief measures include firm support (adhesive strapping or a tight-fitting maternity girdle), heat, and a bed board. Shoes with low or flat heels should be worn to provide a wide base of support.

Reproductive Organ Changes

Apart from uterine changes, the most noticeable changes take place in the vagina and breasts.

Vagina

In preparation for the tremendous elasticity that will be demanded during parturition, the vagina exhibits marked changes during pregnancy. The mucosa thickens, the rugae deepen, smooth muscle cells hypertrophy, and connective tissue softens and loosens. These factors combine to make the birth canal longer and more elastic. When the uterus grows up out of the pelvis, the vagina is pulled upward and lengthened; when lightening takes place, it is pushed back down, which sometimes causes the vaginal wall to fall into horizontal folds.[5] Similarly, the pelvic floor becomes more elastic in preparation for the tremendous distention it will sustain at delivery. The vulva, too, becomes softer, with increased glandular secretions and a characteristic darkening of the mucosa.

Vaginal discharge increases, undoubtedly because of the increased discharge from the endocervical glands, and the **pH** becomes distinctly more acid. It is thought that this acid medium plays a role in reducing the number of pathogenic bacteria present in the vagina. This normal **leukorrhea** has a thick whitish appearance and is nonirritating.

Two common organisms flourish in an acid medium, however: *Candida albicans* (a yeast infection) and *Trichomonas vaginalis. Candidiasis,* also called *moniliasis,* is related to thrush infections in the infant and is frequently present in the vagina without causing symptoms. Women who harbor this infection are sometimes asymptomatic for long periods of time, but the increasingly acid medium of the vagina during pregnancy favors a flare-up. Symptoms include an irritating leukorrhea that causes severe itching of the vulva and external genitalia. The discharge is either thick and yellowish or thin and watery admixed with agglutinated whitish material often described as "cottage cheese."

Trichomonas causes a frothy yellow discharge with intense irritation and itching. It is venereal in origin, and the man with whom the woman has sexual contact should be treated simultaneously. It can be readily identified under the microscope by the characteristic shape of the organism.

Breasts

At **menarche** the immature female breast begins to enlarge until the adult breast, composed of glandular, fatty, and connective tissue, is formed. Thereafter a cyclical engorgement may occur each month under the influence of estrogen. However, breast development cannot be said to be complete until, with pregnancy, the sex hormones estrogen and progesterone interact with the **chorion somatomammotropin** excreted by the placenta. The interaction of these hormones initiates the formation of the alveolar system in the breasts wherein the milk will be formed, and the ductal system, which will transport the milk to the suckling infant.

A cross section of the pregnant or lactating breast shows a well-developed transport system. The nipple, which was pink in the **nullipara,** becomes darker with pregnancy, and the alveolar glands are accentuated. These sebaceous glands in the **areola** look like small pimples; their secretion serves to lubricate and protect the nipple during nursing.

Close examination of the nipple reveals up to 15 separate tiny openings, from which **colostrum** may be expressed in the later months of pregnancy. If we could follow the course of these tiny openings, we would come to saclike enlargements of the duct, which are called lactiferous ducts (or **milk sacs**). These milk sacs will pool the milk. The sucking action of the infant and the pressure of his jaws upon them express the milk forward to the nipple. Following still further back from the nipple, the **lactiferous ducts** branch off into smaller ductules, each of which is surrounded by grapelike clusters called **alveolar lobules.** The milk will eventually be manufactured in these lobules (Fig. 5-7).

After the alveolar and ductal systems have been formed, that is, after about the fifth or sixth month of gestation, colostrum may be found in the breasts. The mother may notice small droplets of colostrum on her nipples and should be instructed to cleanse the nipples with plain water. Soap should not be used to cleanse the nipples in the later months of pregnancy because its drying effect predisposes the nipple to crack during the stress of early nursing.

Because some women, especially those who are fair skinned, experience sore nipples in the early nursing period, many physicians recommend prenatal preparation to condition them. Suggested measures include going without a brassiere for a part of the day or, if the woman is uncomfortable without support for her breasts, cutting a hole in the brassiere to expose the nipple and areola so that friction from clothing accustoms the nipple area to some stress. Gentle massage with a terry washcloth during or after the bath also helps. An emollient such as pure lanolin or baby oil may be applied daily to the areola area, but it should not cover the duct openings. The breasts can be exposed for short periods to ultraviolet rays either from sun in summer or from a sunlamp.

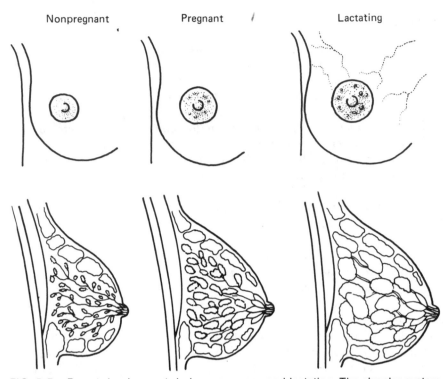

Nonpregnant   Pregnant   Lactating

FIG. 5-7. Breast development during pregnancy and lactation. The alveolar system, where the milk will be produced, and the ductal or transport system are formed and mature under stimulation of the hormones of pregnancy interacting with placental hormones. Beginning close to the chest wall, the alveolar lobules can be seen as grapelike clusters where the milk will be manufactured. Leading toward the nipple through tiny ductules, then into larger lactiferous ducts, eventually the milk pools in saclike enlargements of the lactiferous ducts (milk sacs) behind the areola. The sucking action and the pressure of the infant's jaws bring the milk forward and out through the nipple. (Ross Clinical Education Aid No. 10, The Mammary Glands and Breast Feeding. Columbus, Ross Laboratories)

Another frequent suggestion is rolling or stripping the nipples. The woman can begin doing this twice a day in the eighth month until delivery. First she washes her hands thoroughly. Then she grasps the nipple gently at the outer edge of the areola with the thumb and forefinger of one hand while supporting the breast with the other hand. She then pulls the nipple gently outward toward the tip of the nipple until it just begins to feel uncomfortable. She moves her hand around the nipple gently, rolling and pulling until she has kneaded each area.

The expectant mother needs advice on the purchase of proper brassieres whether or not she plans to nurse. In either case, the brassiere should cover the entire breast and have wide back and shoulder straps. When the brassiere is fitted, the woman should make sure that it is comfortable with the closure at its most snug fastening and that it does not ride up in back when she moves. It should have several rows of hooks to accomodate her change in size when engorgement takes place. The cup should be snug without binding or gaping under the arm.

If the breasts are uncomfortably heavy in late pregnancy or during the **perinatal** period, the woman should wear a brassiere even when sleeping. In this case, the fastening could be at its loosest setting.

If the mother is planning to nurse, a nursing bra should be pruchased with the same criteria in mind. Each cup of a nursing bra opens to allow nursing from one breast, while the other breast is still supported. Plastic liners should be avoided because plastic does not allow the nipples to dry thoroughly, and the increased moisture may lead to itching and irritation of the nipple. If the student has already purchased a brassiere that has a plastic liner and she cannot return it, she should be advised to remove the lining.

If leakage is a concern, a folded, white, ironed man's handkerchief is the ideal liner. The heat of the iron helps to reduce the number of organisms present, and it is absorbent, inexpensive, and ecologically sound because it can be reused. Special nursing pads can be purchased if desired but are in no way superior to the ironed handkerchief. Expectant mothers need to know that leakage will not always be a problem, even if it is at first. Some basic physiology of nursing should be included in your prenatal instructions to give an understanding of the causal relationship between the infant's nursing and the breasts' supply.

Sexual Activity: Controversy and Concern

It helps expectant parents to know something about the normal variations that occur in both eroticism and sexual response during pregnancy. They also need reassurance that their sexual activity is not injurious to the fetus.

Although a very few physicians still interdict sexual intercourse throughout the entire 9 months of gestation, most feel that this not only is unnecessary in the absence of obstetric complications, but also places additional strain on the marriage. Both expectant parents need reassurance that they are loved and desirable in spite of the additional worries or changes in body image that come with pregnancy. The physical expression of that love is extremely important at this time if equilibrium is to be maintained. In their study of 79 husbands of pregnant and puerperal women, Masters and Johnson found that nearly 23% had resorted to extramarital sexual activity during the continence period, many for the first time.[8] At present, medical opinion is still divided about the advisability of interdiction, and those who still routinely advise continence recommend time periods varying from 2 to 8 weeks antenatally.

During the first trimester, many women are not conscious of any change in their sexual desire. Others report a drop in sexual interest, often related to nausea or the general feeling of fatigue in the first trimester. A few, relieved of the need for contraception, enjoy a new feeling of freedom.

The second trimester brings less nausea and, according to some authors, a general rise in sexual feelings for most women, possibly due to pelvic engorgement. Masters and Johnson found that nearly 82% of the women in their sample experienced heightened sexual interest in the middle trimester.[8] This finding was not borne out by Wagner and Solberg, however, who documented a steady decrease in sexual desire and activity throughout pregnancy.[13]

In both studies, sexual activity declined during the third trimester, for various stated reasons. Among them were a decrease in desire due to discomfort or to the woman's "feeling unattractive," fear of harming the fetus, or proscription by the physician. Men in the Masters and Johnson study reported that they were afraid of harming the fetus or their wives. A few found the obvious signs of gestation unappealing.

There appears to be a dearth of information among the general public about sexuality during pregnancy, and many couples hesitate to initiate the subject with their physician. If the physican does not discuss the normalcy of continued sexuality or his rationale for recommending any curtailment of sexual activity, it may make communication between the couple even more difficult. Lacking information, they may assume that sexual activity during pregnancy is improper or shameful. The discomfort experienced in the male-superior position may cause the traditionally minded couple to cease all sexual relations for the duration of the pregnancy. Simple suggestions made by the physician for position change may not only increase their comfort but may also help them accept their own continued sexuality.

A good book that the childbirth educator may wish to recommend to her students is *Making Love During Pregnancy* by Bing and Colman. It is a good source of general information and may be especially helpful to the couple who do not wish to bring the topic up for discussion. (See Appendix C.)

The couple should be informed of signs related to sexual activity that may signal danger and about which they should consult their medical advisor. The most urgent of these is bleeding or spotting after intercourse. The onset of contractions that continue, although not necessarily pathologic, should also be brought to the attention of the physician.

There are several factors in the controversy around sex activity during pregnancy of which the informed childbirth educator should be aware so she can act as a valid resource for her students. Although research into the possible causative relationship between sex activity and premature labor has been conducted and reported for decades, no study has presented clear enough evidence upon which to base any definite conclusions.

Since the time of Hippocrates the fact that orgasm causes the uterus to contract has engendered speculation that it might be a causative factor in premature labor. Research is difficult because the human female is the only known female animal who engages in copulatory activity after impregnation. Although many women experience uterine contractions following orgasm, particularly in the second and third trimesters, Masters and Johnson point out that very few go into premature labor.

There may well be a group who are predisposed to commence labor following orgasm, however. Goodlin, Keller, and Raffin cite several cases in which there was a clear connection between the onset of premature labor and orgasm.[4] In their study they also found that of the puerperas who delivered after 39 weeks' gestation, only 24% were orgasmic after the 32nd week of pregnancy, whereas of the group who delivered prior to 37 weeks' gestation, 50% were orgasmic up until they went into labor. Therefore it would appear that the more orgasmic women were more likely to deliver early.

In another part of their study, they asked five term gravidas who were still orgasmic to achieve orgasm at a specified time to see if labor could be induced. Of the four who were successful, three began labor within 9 hours of orgasm and the fourth had an episode of false labor.

Much interest has been generated lately in the role of the prostaglandins in initiating labor. As early as 1930 it was recognized that the uterus contracted upon the instillation of **semen** into the vagina. By 1935 the active principal was isolated and named *prostaglandin* because of its supposed origin in the prostate. We now know that the uterus, too, produces prostaglandins, which are an active factor in the stimulation of smooth muscle fibers.

As term approaches, the uterus becomes more sensitive to stimulation by the prostaglandins, perhaps because of a decrease in progesterone levels, which allows an increase in myometrial conductivity and excitability. Concomitantly, the level of estrogen rises, increasing vascularity and permeability as well as enhancing rhythmic contractions.[4] It is possible that postorgasmic contractions can be attributed to the increased absorption of prostaglandins from the vagina, which takes place in the presence of the massive vasodilatation that occurs with orgasm.

These hypotheses require further investigation before conclusions can be drawn; however, they do give us some direction in planning for future research. If we can gain insight into the complex interaction of the various agents that initiate labor, we will be ready to do battle with prematurity, our number-one cause of infant deaths.

It is clear that there are no hard and fast rules for the physician to follow when advising the expectant couple about sex activity. In the vast majority of cases there have been no ill effects. Since Masters and Johnson have shown that the uterus responds more strongly to orgasm produced by manipulation than by **coitus,** a fact clearly not accounted for by prostaglandins, an interdiction of intercourse seems pointless in the absence of bleeding, ruptured membranes, or **dyspareunia.** Additional cautions might be indicated in the gravida with a deeply engaged **presenting part** or when the cervix is prematurely ripe. If abortion, miscarriage, or premature labor is threatened, orgasm as well as vaginal intercourse is contraindicated.

The physician must tailor his advice to each individual pregnancy. Active communication between couple and physician is essential. Especially when interdiction must be imposed for some medical consideration, the husband as well as the wife should be informed. Open discussion of alternate measures helps to foster interpersonal concern between husband and wife.

References

1. American College of OB/GYN: Cigarette smoking & pregnancy. ACOG Technical Bulletin 53, Sept 1979
2. Apgar V, Beck J: Is My Baby All Right? p 99. New York, Pocket Books, 1974
3. Crisp WR, DeFranco S: The Hand syndrome of pregnancy. J Obstet Gynecol 23:433, 1964
4. Goodlin RC, Keller DW, Raffin M: Orgasm during late pregnancy: Possible deleterious effects. J Obstet Gynecol 38:6 1971
5. Greenhill JP: Obstetrics, p 176. Philadelphia, WB Saunders, 1965
6. Hellman LM, Pritchard JA: Williams Obstetrics, 14th ed. New York, Appleton-Century-Crofts, 1971
7. Lappe FM: Diet for a Small Planet. New York, Ballantine Books, 1971
8. Masters S, Johnson V: Human Sexual Response, pp 164–165. Boston, Little, Brown & Co, 1966
9. McKay S: Smoking during the childbearing year. Malem Child Nurse J 5, 1980
10. Surgeon General, NICHD: Smoking and infant health. In Surgeon General's Report on Smoking and Health, Chap 8. Rockville, MD, NICDH, 1979
11. Tompkins WT: The clinical significance of nutritional deficiencies in pregnancy. Bull NY Acad Med 24:376–388, 1948
12. Tompkins ST, Wiehl D: Nutritional deficiencies as a causal factor in toxemia and premature labor. Am J Obstet Gynecol 62:898, 1951
13. Wagner N, Solberg D: Pregnancy and sexuality. Medical Aspects of Human Sexuality, March 1974
14. Wiedenbach E: Family Centered Maternity Nursing, 2nd ed, p 220. New York, GP Putnam's Sons, 1967

6

Normal Labor and Delivery

For the **primipara,** lightening takes place about 4 to 6 weeks prior to the expected date of confinement. In the multipara it is more likely to occur closer to term or even after the onset of labor. The mother may notice that the bulge in her body is lower. Some women report that this seems to follow a period of marked intrauterine activity. Subjectively, the mother notes relief of the epigastric pressure and breathlessness caused by indirect pressure aganst the diaphragm and a return of the marked urinary frequency as the bladder is compressed between the uterus and the symphysis pubis. Pressure-related symptoms such as dependent edema and hemorrhoids are often present and are especially pronounced in the multipara.

As the uterus becomes more sensitive to **oxytocin** released from the pituitary, **Braxton Hicks contractions** increase in frequency and become more noticeable. These **contractions** are usually felt mainly in the abdominal area as muscular tightening and relaxation without associated discomfort. There may be periods when they are quite regular in character, causing the mother to speculate that she may be in labor. A change in activity usually causes them to cease, however. Early labor contractions may feel very similar to these, but the parents can differentiate these contractions from labor contractions because the false labor contractions do not progress in terms of length, strength or interval.

In prenatal class, these contractions can be mentioned to acquaint the class with the sensation of a contraction. The childbirth educator reinforces the concept of the body preparing for the work of labor by pointing out what is being accomplished prior to true labor: the cervix softens and becomes "ripe," ready to undergo the changes of labor, as the presenting part moves down into the pelvis; then the cervix swings forward and into the midline. Partial **effacement** may take place, and some **dilatation** is frequently noted in the multipara.

Many women experience a great burst of energy a few days or hours prior to labor. Often referred to as "nesting" by childbirth educators, the expectant mother suddenly has an urge to make the world ready for the expected offspring. She may quite suddenly decide to wash walls, repaint a room, or clean out all the cupboards in her house "before the baby comes." While there is nothing inherently wrong in these activities, the mother should not begin labor in a state of exhaustion. The best advice therefore is "one closet at a time." At least if she empties only one closet, then runs out of energy or goes into labor, it is not a major job to put things back together again. If, on the other hand, she pulls out the contents of every closet in her home, she must either exhaust herself cleaning up or leave everything in a state of chaos.

Avoiding extreme fatigue is an important part of preparing for the work of labor. The body is expected to perform hard physical work for a long period of time under stress. To enable it to do so with optimum efficiency, it must enter the work period well rested and in good physical condition. In supervising prenatal care the physician monitors possible obstetric difficulties, but the expectant mother herself is responsible for following medical advice, eating a healthful diet, preparing herself physically by doing the physical conditioning exercises, and avoiding excessive fatigue.

She should not, of course, sit at home and do nothing! If invited to a late party, she should be encouraged to go if she so desires. However, the importance of making up the missed sleep should be stressed. The effects of a few hours' missed sleep are cumulative, so if she consistently misses even an hour's sleep, over a period of time she will be depleting her energy reserves.

First Stage

Phase I: Latent

Early labor contractions seem to the mother not unlike the increased Braxton Hicks contractions she has experienced in the last few weeks of her pregnancy. They may center more in the back, the sensation radiating around to the front. Over a period of time these contractions become longer, stronger, and closer together. A change of activity does not cause them to stop. The parents can be told to look for these characteristics and to time the contractions for at least an hour before reporting that labor has begun. Ruptured membranes or any abnormality such as bleeding or very rapidly progressing contractions should be reported immediately.

Physiology

The latent phase should not last longer than about 20 hours in the nulliparous woman or 14 hours in the multipara. This phase may be prolonged, however, by an "unripe" cervix or injudicious use of sedation as well as pathologic factors such as myometrial dysfunction, which results in desultory labor.

During this preparatory time the cervix is getting ready for the change in the dilatation phase. If effaces and begins early dilatation. Usually the onset of labor is considered the commencement of more or less regular and progressive contractions as perceived by the mother. This rather subjective reckoning remains the usual criterion because physiologists are unable to differentiate scientifically between contractions that will progress into active labor and those that will cease. The early labor contractions are erratic, and the myometrial contraction wave is less coordinated than it will become. As labor progresses, the contraction wave becomes stronger in the upper third of the fundus, shortening myometrial fibers in the upper fundus so that following each contraction the upper fundus is infinitesimally thicker. As this occurs there is a corresponding thinning of the cervix. The muscle tonus remains the same in the interval between contractions.

Generally, the contractions last about 30 to 45 sec, beginning rather irregularly, but becoming more regular as they become more coordinated. They may begin 15 or 20 min apart or closer, and the gravida may notice some blood-tinged or pink mucous discharge, which is the mucous plug. By the end of the latent phase, the contractions may be around 5 min apart, lasting 55 to 60 sec (Fig. 6-1). In terms of work accomplished, the cervix has effaced and has begun to dilate to around 2 to 3 cm (Fig. 6-2).

The contractions should be timed, but parents need not time them all.

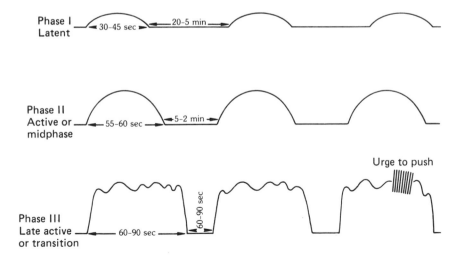

FIG. 6-1. Contraction chart suitable for use in expectant parents' classes. This chart, simply reproduced by the childbirth educator, can be used to depict the wavelike character and changing intensity of the contractions during the first stage of labor.

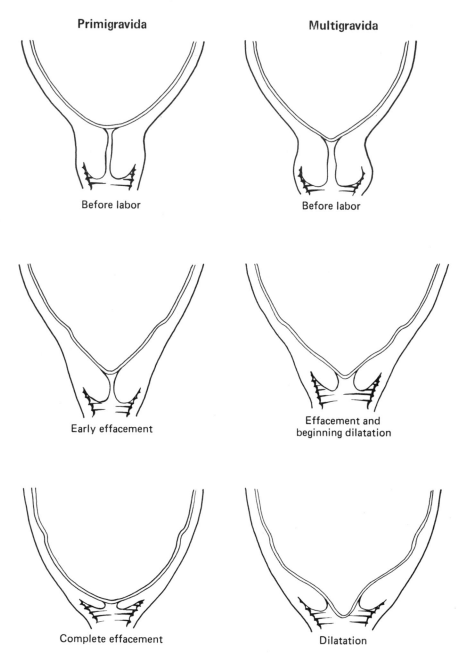

Primigravida

Multigravida

Before labor

Before labor

Early effacement

Effacement and
beginning dilatation

Complete effacement

Dilatation

FIG. 6-2. Cervical effacement and dilatation. The primiparous cervix is more resistant than the multiparous cervix, effacing and dilating slowly over a period of many hours. In the multipara, the cervix is frequently partially effaced and dilated before the onset of labor; the dilatation proceeds more rapidly. (Ross Clinical Education Aid No. 13, Cervical Effacement and Dilatation. Columbus, Ross Laboratories, 1973)

Too many women in very early labor enter the hospital already fatigued by hours of concentration on contractions. They can be instructed to time a few; then, unless some obvious change occurs, forget about timing for a while. After an hour or so, time a few more to see if there has been any progress.

Care of the Mother

During most of the latent phase the woman usually remains out of the hospital. To be prepared for this waiting time, expectant couples need a clear idea of what they should expect in terms of contractions, mood, and the work that is being accomplished. They also need to be aware of deviations from the normal pattern so that they know when to call the physician.

The best advice for the woman in very early labor is to take a nap or go back to sleep if it is night. Unfortunately this advice is nearly impossible to follow because of the excitement of being in labor at last. The next best thing is for her to entertain herself in some way other than by timing contractions. If it is during the day, the labor coach might suggest some diverting and unfatiguing activity such as a movie.

During this phase of labor, the mother is often ambivalent. She may have been eagerly looking forward to the day when she would go into labor, yet, when it arrives she is almost afraid to believe it is true. Not infrequently, in telling the story of her labor, the new mother will recall that she thought it was false labor and would go away. Her dependency needs, which have been increasing throughout the prenatal period, become more evident as labor begins and continue to increase throughout **parturition.** She wants to be sure that those she has been counting on to help at this time will be with her throughout labor.

The labor coach's task during this time is to help the mother keep calm and to surround her with a supportive atmosphere. He can suggest entertainment or offer to take care of any last-minute tasks. He can provide distractions to keep her from beginning to use her respiratory techniques for labor before they are necessary.

To preserve the option of general anesthesia, the obstetrician may prohibit eating once labor has begun. Gastric motility, already retarded during pregnancy, slows down further during labor, thus increasing the time it takes to empty the stomach contents. This makes the danger of aspiration very real when inhalation anesthesia is used because it abolishes the reflex that otherwise prevents regurgitation. Furthermore, a full stomach causes the mother discomfort during labor and may well be the cause of vomiting during the transitional phase.

The mother still needs fluids and a level of blood sugar adequate for her body's energy needs. Some obstetricians routinely order an intravenous infusion on all patients in labor. If inhalation anesthesia is not contemplated or if the obstetrician has not prohibited any intake at all, the mother should be instructed to limit her intake to fluids or clear fluids. Since fats and milk solids are likely to remain in the stomach longer, she would be wise to avoid dairy products. Tea, well sweetened with honey, is an ideal supplier of both fluid and energy.

A warm shower or, if the membranes are not ruptured, a bath, may give her a feeling of well-being and help her to relax.

One way to facilitate a smooth transition from home to the hospital is to check out the route to the hospital, with alternatives, well in advance of labor. The expectant parents should locate parking facilities, the appropriate entrance to the hospital, etc. If possible, the mother should preregister, taking her health insurance card with her and answering the necessary questions when she is not under the stress of labor. If a regular tour of the obstetric unit is offered, the childbirth educator should by all means encourage them to go. This assists them in structuring their concept of labor and makes it more real to them.

Phase II: Accelerated (or Active)

Physiology

The latent phase ends with the cervix completely effaced and dilated to about 2 to 3 cm. The contractions change in character and become more clearly defined, with a more definite increment, peak, and decrement. At the beginning of the accelerated phase, they last about 55 to 60 sec, with about a 2-min interval (see Fig. 6-1). During this phase, the myometrial activity accelerates to dilate the cervix actively. Because the contractions differ in character, for teaching purposes we may divide this accelerated phase into two sections: the active phase (*i.e.*, the period of maximum slope on the Friedman graph, or from 4-8 cm) and the transitional phase (corresponding to the deceleration phase on the graph, or from 8-10 cm in terms of cervical dilatation; Fig. 6-3). Concurrently, the presenting part is moving down.

During the active or accelerated phase, the contractions are well defined and fall into a definite pattern. Although most women experience regular contractions, a few never establish a regular rhythm. Their pattern may have an irregular rhythm, such as a strong contraction, 4-min interval, mild contraction, 2-min interval, strong contraction, 4-min interval, and so forth. Usually each contraction closely resembles the one that preceded it, with a peak of about 30 sec.

Hospital Admission

The prepared woman is usually quite businesslike when admitted to the hospital. Gone is the bubbly, excited mood that was characteristic of

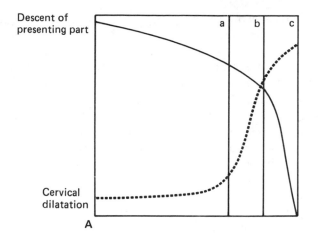

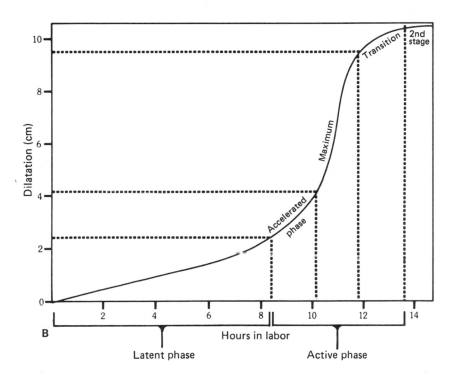

FIG. 6-3. Friedman labor graphs. (*A*) The rate of descent of the presenting part compared with cervical dilatation during the latent phase (*a*), dilatation (*b*), and pelvic or second stage (*c*) of labor. (*B*) The average rate of cervical dilatation during the latent phase, active phase, and second stage of labor. (Friedman EA: The functional divisions of labor. Am J Obstet Gynecol 104:274–280, 1971)

early labor; it has been replaced with a more workmanlike quality. The contractions have started and are fairly consistent so that she knows she will be able to cope with the next one much as she was able to cope with the last. If fatigue is not too great a factor, her coping mechanisms are well activated and she is likely to feel quite proud of how well she is doing. She is usually well oriented to place, although her time sense is distorted. It may seem to her that she has been in labor forever, but when told the time, she expresses disbelief that so much time has elapsed. Her ego boundaries are still fairly secure at this point, and although she may request medication for pain relief if she is unable to relax effectively, there is a general sense of being in control.

The woman is usually admitted to the labor room during this accelerated phase and prepared for delivery according to her physician's orders. This usually, but not invariably, includes a shaving or clipping of some of the perineal hair and an enema. A history is taken of the course of labor, and the woman is asked if membranes are intact. She has an initial admission vaginal exam and should ask about her dilatation if this information is not offered spontaneously. Her blood pressure, pulse, and fetal heart are monitored. She receives some type of identification band with a tiny one attached that is to be placed on her infant in the delivery room. In addition, she may be asked for a urine sample and blood may be taken. If the hospital's or physician's routine for labor includes an intravenous infusion or placing the mother on the fetal monitor, it is done at this time.

Followng the admission procedure, the woman and her labor coach settle down to the business of timing contractions. The coach jots down the time and length of each contraction. As each one begins, signaled by the parturient's deep **signal breath,** he calls off 15-sec intervals to help circumscribe the time for her. He also looks for signs of tension and signals its release with the tactile and verbal cues for controlled relaxation they have practiced in the preparatory period (see Appendix A). If the rate of her respiration becomes too fast or she loses her focus of concentration, he can help her to get back on the track by breathing with her, with his face directly in her line of vision for a few contractions.

Other comfort measures include those things that the labor room nurse would ordinarily do in the absence of a labor coach: suggesting positional changes, suggesting that the bladder be emptied hourly, coaxing and comforting and providing a supportive environment.

Phase III: Transition (or Late Active)

Physiology

The time termed *transition* marks the end of the first stage, with the cervix dilating 8 to 10 cm. This has been called deceleration by Friedman, because progress seems to slow down if measured solely in terms of cervical dilatation (see Fig. 6-3). As the graphs show, this is misleading. The dilatation appears to slow down because progress is now occurring in the downward movement of the presenting part. If they are not to become discouraged, parents need to know that progress is measured not only in terms of cervical dilatation, but also in terms of station. The transition phase lasts roughly 30 to 60 min in the primipara, 20 to 30 min in the multipara, and even less as parity increases.

The contractions last about 60 to 90 sec if the labor is not being stimulated with oxytocin, with a 60- to 90-sec interval. For the first time, it is possible that the contraction will last longer than the rest period. The contractions rise sharply, usually peaking within a few seconds of onset. The peak itself is irregular, giving a sense of turbulence to the contraction (see Fig. 6-1). The sensation is similar to that experienced when one lifts something too heavy; the muscles shake violently under the strain. To add to the difficulties, the contractions are no longer very regular, but keep coming on before the mother has had an opportunity to catch her breath from the preceding one.

Other symptoms of transition include an increase in bloody show, trembling of the limbs, increasing back pressure (as the presenting part moves down in the pelvis), and cold extremities.

Care of the Mother

A marked increase in body language may be observed, as the mother psychologically withdraws into herself. She is so totally involved with what is going on within her own body that she is less able to articulate or even formulate her needs. Her verbal language becomes more childlike, her sentences more fragmented. Suggestions must be made in short, clear sentences, for she does not have the energy to carry on a conversation. It is at this time particularly that she must be able to lean on her labor coach. He must provide active and constant support, talking her through each contraction (what one obstetrician has termed "verbal analgesia"). She needs continuous encouragement and reinforcement, and she needs to be told that she is doing well, and that soon she will be able to push and will feel much better.

For most women, the transition phase is the most difficult part of labor. The contractions are long, strong, and very nearly overwhelming. No matter how successful the woman has been at staying relaxed during her labor, the rigors of several hours of hard muscular activity have left her fatigued and irritable. Her withdrawal from interaction with others leaves her feeling somewhat isolated and helpless in the face of the awesome force of the contractions. Small wonder she is likely to become whiny and complaining. Her desire to escape from the rest of the labor is reflected in her efforts to fall asleep between contractions or in a stated, if irrational, desire to "forget it." She may say she doesn't want a baby . . . or to the husband, "You finish up here, I'm going home!" Feeling unable to face many more of these relentless contractions, she may demand to be put to sleep. *It is essential that she be told of her progress and that the end is near.*

It is important that she remain alert at this time. Because of the shortened interval between contractions and the rapid peaking of the contractions, she must be ready to begin her technique right at the start of the contraction, before it is so strong that she cannot cope with it. The labor coach can help by refreshing her with a cool washcloth, sponging her face and neck. If she is attached to the fetal monitor, the coach can give her a verbal cue when the contraction begins to show on the graph.

Because the diaphragm is getting ready for the urge to bear down, the woman may feel somewhat queasy. She may belch and in some cases vomit. Just before the woman feels the need to push, the labor coach may observe a slight expiratory grunt. This is followed, in a contraction or two, by the definite desire to close the **glottis** and bear down. This is the time to ask for an examination. Even if one has been done fairly recently, the urge to push is a signal that things are changing, and it is important for the couple to know exactly where the woman is in her labor so that they can assess appropriate responses.

The primiparous woman must not bear down before she has been examined and given permission. Pushing against a cervix that is not fully dilated may result in an edematous cervix, which will cause further problems. In the multiparous patient there is also the possibility that her efforts will lead to a precipitate delivery. In order to prevent premature pushing, she may be instructed to change her respiratory pattern to a series of short staccato puff-blows. This puff-blow exhalation can be accomplished only by sharply raising the diaphragm, thus making it impossible to lower the diaphragm to bear down (see Appendix A). When permitted to push, the woman partially closes her glottis, blocking the air in her lungs, relaxes the **key areas** (*i.e.*, jaw and perineum), and bears down with her diaphragm and abdominal muscles.

Fortunately, although transition is the hardest part of labor, it is also the shortest and signals the end of the long first stage. Once the cervix is fully dilated and the woman begins to bear down effectively, she feels tremendously relieved and anxious to get on with it. When teaching about the transition phase, the childbirth teacher can stress these positive aspects so that it can be put into perspective by the couple. It will not seem frightening if it can be viewed as a sign of real progress.

Second Stage

A simple overview of the mechanics of labor early in the class series will lay the groundwork for a return to the subject in more detail later, when the teacher is ready to talk about the second stage in terms of contractions, mood, sensations, techniques, and coaching role (Table 6-1). The object of an early introduction of labor is to build a general framework so that the couple has a feeling of preparedness.

The first stage of labor saw the uterine contents overcoming the soft tissue resistance, with the resultant dilatation of the cervix and lower uterine segment. The upper portion of the vagina, which is attached to the cervix, becomes dilated also, resulting in a birth canal that is tunnel shaped. By the second stage, the membranes are usually ruptured so that the presenting part becomes the dilating force. As the contractions continue to exert pressure from above, the baby is moved downward in the direction of least resistance. Voluntarily the mother aids the force of the contractions by exerting downward pressure with the diaphragm and abdominal muscles. This expulsive effort becomes involuntary as the presenting part moves lower and comes into contact with the muscles of the pelvic floor. These contractions last about 65 to 90 sec, but unlike the transition period, there is an interval of several minutes between contractions, giving the mother a short rest period.

Diagrams or a model of a pelvis will show the class that the transverse diameter of the female pelvis is slightly longer than its anterior–posterior diameter. The instructor can use diagrams or even show on her own head that the head, too, has a long and a short diameter (Fig. 6-4). After this demonstration, the discussion logically turns to the rotations that the fetus must make in order to negotiate the pelvic inlet, true pelvis, and pelvic floor in the process of birth.

The baby enters the pelvis at right angles to the plane of the pelvic inlet. As the presenting part meets with resistance, flexion forces the fetal chin back against the fetal chest, thus presenting the smallest possible diameter at the inlet (occipitofrontal to suboccipitobregmatic; Fig. 6-5). In over 60% of patients, the head is in a transverse position at the onset of labor, that is, the long diameter of the head fitting into the long axis of the pelvis.

As descent occurs and the fetal head reaches the level of the **ischial spines** (Fig. 6-6), it rotates to face the mother's back (occasionally it rotates to face anteriorly). The greatest diameter of the pelvis is now anteroposterior, due to encroachment of the ischial spines. The occiput now comes under the lower rim of the symphysis, which acts as a fulcrum when the resistance of the perineal muscles exerts pressure anteriorly, causing extension of the fetal head.

The head is born by extension, with the crown appearing first at the vaginal opening, and the perineum then slipping back over the baby's face (with or without an episiotomy) so that the eyes, nose, then chin appear as the head is born. Once the head is free, it rotates again to be in line with the rest of the fetal body still within the pelvis.

Although the fetal head is the largest part to negotiate the pelvis, the

(Text continues on p 100)

Table 6-1. **Labor Summary**

Stage or Phase of Labor	Contractions	Progress	Parturient's Mood	Techniques Employed	Coaching Role
Stage I					
Early labor	Mild, 35–45 sec duration, 20–5 min intervals	Cervix effaces and dilates to 2–3 cm	Excited to be in labor at last; somewhat ambivalent	None or controlled relaxation as necessary; avoid fatigue	Entertain the parturient. Keep her from beginning her techniques too soon. Prepare for transition to the hospital. Provide a calm atmosphere.
Accelerated (early active)	Becoming more definite, 45–60 sec duration, 5–2½ min intervals	Cervix dilates 2–8 cm; presenting part moves down in pelvis	Businesslike, concentrates well with contractions; may tire toward end; begins to wonder about own ability to remain in control	(1) **Rhythmic chest breathing**, (2) modified **RCB**, (3) combined rhythm, accelerated/decelerated rhythm for emergencies (see Appendix A)	Time contractions and count off seconds. Watch for tension and signal its release. Provide encouragement and comfort measures. Remind her to empty bladder.
Transition (late active)	Tremendously strong, peaking rapidly and repeatedly, 60–90 sec duration, 60–90 sec interval	Cervix dilates 8–10 cm	Withdrawn, wants to give up; irritable, fatigued, difficulty in relaxing between contractions; increase in body language; increase in show, back pressure; trembling limbs; may experience urge to push down	Puff-blow rhythm, blow out for urge to push; controlled relaxation or rhythmic chest breathing between contractions; concentration on getting through to the next puff	Employ the same measures as above, plus constant strong encouragement. Keep her informed of progress. Remind her that the end of the first stage is near. Tell her how well she is doing. Support her lower back. Breathe with her if she loses the rhythm. Count the breathing rhythm for her. Stroke, coax, comfort!

Stage	Contractions		Emotional/Behavioral	Breathing	Support Measures
Stage II Expulsion	Strong, more than 1 min duration, 1-2 min interval	Baby moves down through birth canal and is born	Refreshed, working hard with contractions, strongly positive emotions late in second stage	Pushing Relax and blow out	Initiate pushing activity with verbal cues. Support shoulders or legs as necessary. Watch direction of push. **Remind her to take a full breath before pulling up to push. Remind her to relax key areas.** Reinforce the physician's or midwife's directions by repeating into her ear. **Remind her to stop pushing when instructed for controlled birth of the head.**
Stage III Placental	Mild	Placenta expelled	Relieved, joyful, excited; wants to "claim" infant immediately; needs to hold, stroke, smell and identify newborn May initiate breast-feeding if desired	Push for placenta	Share your joy and excitement with the new mother. If you are the father, you too should hold the infant and count fingers and toes, *etc.*

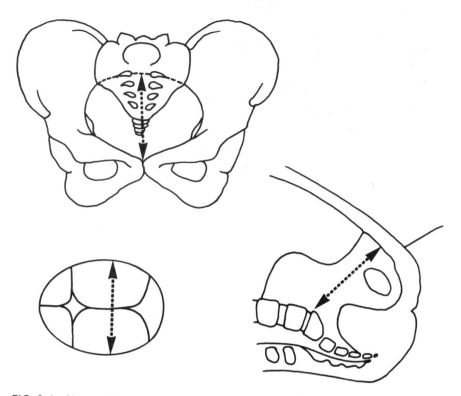

FIG. 6-4. Narrow diameters of the pelvis and the fetal skull. The infant must negotiate the bony pelvis by rotating so that the long axis of the head and the long axis of the shoulders fit down through the long axis of the pelvis. (Modified from Ross Clinical Education Aid No. 13, Mechanisms of Normal Labor. Columbus, Ross Laboratories, 1973)

shoulders likewise have a long and a short axis and follow the pathway of the head in negotiating the planes of the pelvis. As the head is born, the shoulders are coming underneath the symphysis, rotating to accomodate to the larger anteroposterior diameter. Externally, the head rotates laterally, in the direction opposite from the one taken in the internal rotation. As the obstetrician or midwife supports the infant's head, the next few contractions bring about the birth of the anterior shoulder, then the posterior shoulder, and the rest of the baby slides quickly out.

The mother's physical sensations during the second stage vary widely and are strongly influenced by the way she feels about participation or nonparticipation in the birth. If she is frightened of the sensations and wishes not to participate, she may find the contractions unbearable, tensing her voluntary muscles and fighting the descent of the baby against the pelvic floor with all her strength.

Most women women who are not frightened and who can analyze their

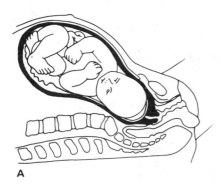
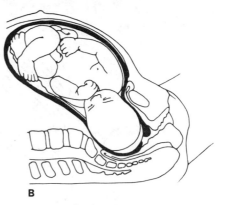

A

B

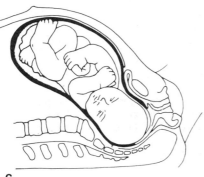
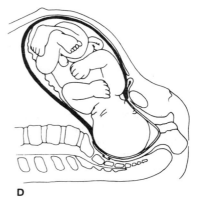

C

D

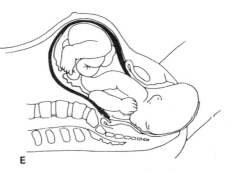

E

FIG. 6–5. Mechanism of normal labor: first and second stages. The cervix effaces and dilates as the fetus descends through the pelvis, rotating to accommodate the bony pelvis. As the head comes under the symphysis, the crown appears at the introitus and the head is born by extension. The shoulders then rotate around the symphysis and are born. The second stage is complete as the infant slides out. (Birth Atlas, 6th ed. New York, Maternity Center Association, 1975)

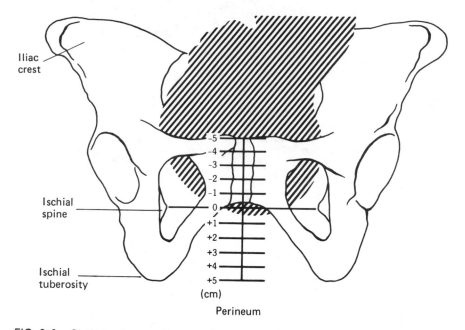

Iliac
crest

Ischial
spine

Ischial
tuberosity

(cm)

Perineum

FIG. 6–6. **Stations** of presenting part. The degree of engagement is measured by the location of the presenting part in the relation to the ischial spines. When the presenting part has reached the level of the ischial spines it is expressed as station 0; above the level of the ischial spines it is measured in minus centimeters; below the level of the ischial spines it is expressed as plus centimeters. Plus 5 cm is the level of the perineum. (Ross Clinical Education Aid No. 13, Mechanism of Normal Labor. Columbus, Ross Laboratories, 1973)

sensations report tremendous pressure and a stretching, burning sensation in the birth canal. When the head is low enough to impinge against the perineum, the mother feels a momentary splitting sensation as the perineum is stretched, then numbness. The childbirth educator may explain this numbness in terms of pressure of the fetal head against the nerves that supply the perineum. An alternative way of phrasing this is to describe how the baby moves down as the mother pushes with the contraction, then slips back as she relaxes. However, when the presenting part is so far down that the symphysis prevents its slipping back, the perineum stretches out instead. This can be put into positive terms by stressing that if the head is so low, it will probably be born with the next contraction. The labor coach should be forewarned that, although up until now his wife has been pushing away with all her strength, the momentary stretching sensation may take her by surprise and cause her to cry out. He should be instructed to remind her that this means the baby is almost here and perhaps to look for **crowning.**

Just at this point, the woman may be instructed to stop pushing so that the outlet can gradually adjust to the pressure of the presenting part. This can reduce overstretching of the perineum and the possibility of tearing. In this case, the parturient should lie back and use controlled relaxation, panting gently through an open mouth.

Subjectively, the second stage is a relief after the difficult transition phase. The fact that the mother is at last able to do something to hasten the birth makes her feel less helpless. Strongly positive feelings occur, especially late in the second stage, for prepared mothers. In spite of the sensations of tremendous stretching and pressure, most women report significantly less pain during the second stage as long as they are bearing down during the contractions. Others report that, although they experienced some pain, they felt they could cope with it.

The childbirth educator needs to beware of giving the impression that, because the second stage feels better than the transition phase, it is easy. Parents need to be prepared for the hard physical labor that is involved. The mother has a renewed sense of purpose, a second wind; at the same time she is working harder than she will ever again until she has another child.

The second stage is a busy time for the labor coach. He signals the start of pushing by the verbal cues (perhaps lifting the parturient's shoulders or legs), directs her work effort, and watches the direction of push. In the interval between contractions, he encourages her to rest, sponges her face and neck, offers ice chips. His constant encouragement is augmented now by encouragement from the labor room nurse and the physician, as they "cheer on" the pushing effort.

The nulliparous woman is usually allowed to push in the labor room until the baby's head begins to show. The multipara is likely to be moved to the delivery room when she begins to push.

Parents should be told what the baby's head will look like when it makes its first appearance at the **introitus.** The vaginal opening gapes with the pushing as the infant moves down in the pelvis, then the perineum begins to bulge and the crown appears. Parents who are unprepared are horrified to observe a wet, wrinkled, bluish object in no way resembling their conception of a baby's head. A verbal description, a film, or slides can help prepare parents for the appearance of the infant's scalp when the head is still under pressure in the birth canal.

Third Stage

As the baby exits from the uterus and the uterus continues to contract, the placental site becomes smaller than the placenta and it begins to come away from the uterine wall. Usually about 10 min after delivery of the infant, the placenta is fully detached and waiting to be delivered (Fig. 6–7). The obstetrician knows it is time to deliver the placenta both by the

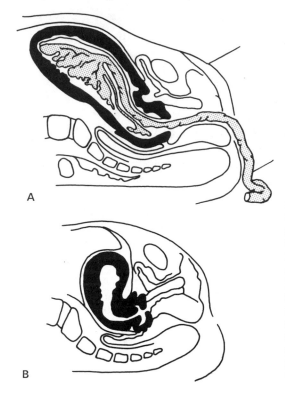

A

B

FIG. 6–7. (A) After the baby is delivered, the uterus continues to contract and the placenta is squeezed out of the uterine lining. About 10–20 min after delivery of the infant the placenta is usually detached and ready to be expelled. (B) After delivery of the placenta the placental site is a raw open wound. The uterus must continue to contract firmly to avoid excessive bleeding. (Birth Atlas, 6th ed. New York, Maternity Center Association, 1975)

globular shape of the uterus and by the fact that the cord suddenly elongates. The mother may then be instructed to bear down again, or fundal pressure may be applied. The obstetrician then examines the placenta carefully to be certain that it is whole, that no parts that may lead to hemorrhage are retained. Should he feel that part of the placenta has been retained, the mother is put to sleep for the few minutes it takes to perform a manual removal or curettage. The couple should be prepared for this eventuality because knowing about the possibility in advance helps to keep its importance in proportion for the few to whom it happens. The mother wakes up a few minutes later; the baby is still there, and it should not seriously mar her memory of the delivery.

Following the expulsion of the placenta, a vaginal exam is usually done to ascertain if there are any tears in the cervix, vaginal vault, or vagina. This exam is fairly uncomfortable for the mother, who needs support from those around her to help her return to her breathing technique if necessary or to provide distraction. The episiotomy is then repaired if one was done, after which the legs are released from the stirrups and brought down gently. A perineal pad is applied, and the fundus is palpated to detect signs of relaxation that might result in unnecessary bleeding. Fundal massage may be done by the nurses, or they may show the mother how to do it.

Meanwhile, the parents' attention is all on their newborn. If the mother has not had much sedation, the infant may cry as soon as the head is free, or this may be delayed for several seconds. Parents need to be prepared for the infant's appearance, which may not be what they expect if they have never seen a newborn before. **Moulding** of the head, vernix, and skin color should all be explained prior to the birth if possible. The cyanotic appearance of the infant before it has drawn its first postnatal breath may frighten the parents. They are less likely to fear for their child if they are aware that the increase in CO_2 that causes the bluish color also stimulates the respiratory center.

While the mother is in the third stage of her labor, the infant is held head downward to promote drainage from the airway. If it is not breathing spontaneously, its back is gently stimulated. The airway is suctioned. The cord is clamped and cut when it has stopped pulsating, and the infant is placed either on its mother's stomach or on a nearby table where the physician or midwife can quickly examine it for gross abnormalities. The Apgar score is taken. The labor room nurse then removes the infant, places it in a heated crib in slight Trendelenburg's position to promote drainage, and follows the hospital's routine in identifying the newborn, instilling medication into the eyes, and so forth. Follow-up on the initial 1-min Apgar score is done at 5 min and again at 15 min. The infant is then wrapped in a warmed receiving blanket and, hospital rules permitting, handed to its parents to hold for the first time.

Integration of Knowledge

It is not enough to offer information. In preparing for a stressful situation such as labor, the childbirth educator must help the couple to integrate their knowledge into their coping systems.

The fact that the expectant parents have come to class does not necessarily indicate that they are both convinced that they will "go through with it" when the time comes. We are a society of students; we take courses to learn how to repair our homes, to take or paint a picture, to have a baby. As the reality of the labor approaches, there is frequently a tendency for the couple to intellectualize the whole event. This is a distancing mechanism, an attempt to solve the problem of labor intellectually without admitting its physical aspects. Typically, the person who reacts in this way is well read and asks the most profound of questions. When it comes to actually practicing techniques, however, little effort is demonstrated.

The instructor's task is to make clear the reality of the coming labor. If the techniques for labor are to be helpful, the woman must use the disciplines of practice so that conditioning can occur. The techniques are still physiologically sound without conditioning, but they cannot fully accomplish their purpose. Without conditioning, the woman will need to think through her responses with each contraction and direct her body to comply. This is fatiguing and unpredictable.

One teaching approach is to have the couple perform the techniques in class and to ask the labor coach how the woman has been doing in her practice. This reinforces the team concept and gives the coach the responsibility of observing her practice and performance.

Sometimes the couple disagree about how a particular technique should be done. Rather than correcting or taking sides, the childbirth instructor should remind them of the criteria for judgment and allow them to reach their own conclusions. This is a first step toward problem solving for labor. For example, if John Smith thinks that Mary Smith is not doing her respiratory techniques correctly, the instructor might begin by asking him what he sees as the problem. If he feels that she is tense, the instructor might place the responsibility right back on him by asking how he will go about helping her to be less tense. If he feels that her exhalation is too long, the class might discuss what would happen if the exhalations are longer than the inhalations. What would the symptoms be? What would it lead to? How can the labor coach help to correct this problem? This type of approach is far more valuable to the class than giving them the correct answer, because it elicits their participation.

The couple should use role playing during each of their practice periods, imagining an actual contraction occuring rather than just going through the motions.

Many instructors use role playing to encourage and observe problem solving in an imaginary labor situation. The class labor rehearsal should be well thought out in advance and should cover unexpected situations. Many students may not really believe that the contraction may occur before they are ready. For this reason, the labor rehearsal should include such possibilities as a contraction during the enema or while being pushed down the hall to the delivery room. These are also situations that require the coach to use his knowledge to try to find a way to make his wife comfortable. Some couples are able to perform well during a class labor rehearsal, others less well, but all can benefit from thinking through the possibilities.

Another approach that can demonstrate the physical aspect of labor is to use a discomfort signal during practice contractions. While the parturient is consciously releasing her voluntary muscles and concentrating on her respiratory responses, the coach applies pressure, gradually increasing it during the **increment** to about 15 to 20 sec. Over the peak of the contraction he maintains the pressure and then, after about 45 sec, gradually decreases the pressure during the **decrement.** He can apply this pressure either on the thigh over the rectus femoris or, if the woman suffers from varicosities, on the Achilles tendon. The woman adjusts her breathing to the strength of the "contraction" and practices keeping the rest of her body relaxed. Simultaneously the coach watches for signs of tension (muscle tightening, clenched jaw, wrinkled brow, *etc.*) and signals their release. This demonstration can be turned into an excellent example of the efficacy of the technique if the coach, immediately after the practice contraction, applies the pressure again as he did at the peak of the contraction. This usually results in cries of amazement at the difference in perception when the woman is no longer concentrating on her technique.

Movies of prepared couples coping with childbirth, as well as slides, are valuable adjuncts to a childbirth preparation program. It should be emphasized that the birth portrayed on film will not be identical to their own birth experience, however.

In choosing appropriate films it is best to look for one that approximates the situation that the class will find as closely as possible. The instructor should view it personally so that she can anticipate questions and frame her responses appropriately. A current descriptive list of films is available in the International Childbirth Education Association (ICEA) Film Directory and may be ordered from their Supplies Center (see Appendix C). Many films are available free or for a moderate fee applicable toward the purchase price.

Labor and delivery slides may be used if a film is not available. The advantage of slides is that, while they are not as exciting as a film, they can be interrupted at any time to point out facts that the instructor feels are important or to answer questions.

Several of the pharmaceutical companies publish booklets for teaching expectant parents. They include some excellent pictures that show moulding, vernix, **milia,** and so forth, and are especially helpful in preparing parents for the appearance of their infant. A thorough description of the infant, including irregular breathing patterns, the relative size of various parts, characteristics of the early neonatal period, appearance of the head, eyes, cord, and so forth encourages expectant parents to think about the infant as a reality.

Labor reports from previous students also help integrate knowledge (Appendix B). If the labor reports are candid in reporting difficulties and how the couple managed to cope with them, they reinforce the idea of preparing for the unexpected. Reading about the unlimited variations of labor helps keep the expectant couple from presupposing what their exact experience will be and encourages flexibility.

The childbirth educator may elect to use some or all of these suggestions for increasing the integration of knowledge. She must keep in mind that the goal is to help the couple become knowledgeable participants in the labor process, capable of assessing and adapting their responses to the demands of labor. Some class groups respond well to discussion approaches; others need more visual aides. The instructor must adapt her presentation to fulfill the specific needs of each group.

7

Preparation for Variations of Labor

First Stage

Posterior Labor

The most common variation of first stage labor is posterior labor or "back" labor, that is, a labor in which the woman experiences most of the discomfort in her back. The back pain is usually described as a dull aching or boring sensation that may not completely disappear between contractions. The incidence is about 30% of all labors.

The most common cause of back pain is a posterior presentation with the hard **occiput** pressing against the maternal structures, bone, muscle, or ligament. It is easy for expectant parents to understand that, since a posterior rotation is not ideal for negotiating the pelvis and birth canal, there may be changes in the pattern of labor. Because the fetal head does not fit down snugly against the soft tissues, a longer, less regular labor pattern may evolve.

If the fetus rotates by the end of the first stage, there is an immediate termination of the backache symptoms, and a more usual second stage ensues. If it does not rotate, the physician or midwife may try a forceps rotation to favor a quicker descent or may wait to see if the mother can rotate it herself with her pushing efforts. Some have found this occurs more readily if the mother pushes in the all-fours position. Sometimes the infant is delivered in the posterior position.

There are four major categories of comfort measures that couples can try for back labor. They are position, pressure, controlled relaxation, and temperature.

Position

The laboring woman who is experiencing back pain should choose a position that allows the weight of the fundus and baby to fall away from her back. She may choose a lateral position with the weight of the fundus resting on the bed. Alternatively, she might choose a high Fowler's position with her back rounded slightly, her elbows resting on her knees and a support behind the sacrum. The instructor and her students can be creative in imagining various positions as long as it is understood that they should be nonstressful and keep the weight of the fundus forward.

During labor the position should be changed at least every half hour, partly because this avoids fatiguing any one body part and improves circulation and partly because motion seems to stimulate the labor and encourage rotation of the baby. In between position changes the mother can get up on all fours and do some rhythmic pelvic tilting as she has learned to do in prenatal class (see Appendix A).

Keeping the pelvis in an anterior tilt position is important to maintain comfort. The woman herself may do pelvic tilting in the lateral position, or the labor coach may do it for her. The coach stands in front of the parturient, places one hand on the anterior superior iliac crest and presses upward. With the other he reaches over her and presses firmly downward against the area where she feels the discomfort. The pressures can be alternated to achieve a passive pelvic tilt (Fig. 7–1).

The couples must be encouraged to practice the suggested positions for back labor if they are to integrate these positions into their repertoire for labor. There is a tendency to assume that it "won't happen to me," which makes it worthwhile to have couples practice their breathing techniques in a back labor position in at least one class practice session.

Pressure

Counterpressure applied over the lumbosacral area can help to equalize the pressure caused by the descent of the presenting part. Most women report that the more firmly pressure is applied, the more relief is afforded. Labor coaches should be reassured that they will not harm the baby or the mother by pushing firmly.

The pressure can be applied in a number of ways. All of them should be

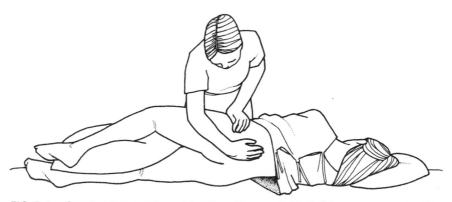

FIG. 7–1. Coach doing passive pelvic tilting. The coach exerts firm pressure against the coccyx with the heel of his hand while pulling posteriorly against the upper superior iliac crest. Pressures may be alternated to achieve a passive pelvic tilt.

practiced in the prenatal period so that the couple will have alternatives to choose from in labor. The woman may be in lying on her side with the coach either in front of her and applying pressure as described in passive pelvic tilting or behind her and applying pressure with the heel of his hand to the place where she feels the discomfort. The exact location for pressure differs from labor to labor and moves downward as the fetus descends through the pelvis. In order to avoid pushing the parturient over on to her abdomen or off the bed, the coach's other hand can rest on the upper iliac crest to stabilize her position. The coach can also apply pressure with his two fists to the area of discomfort, massage the area with his fingertips to increase sensory input, or grasp the two iliac crests with his fingertips and use the thumbs to massage firmly.

Mechanical aids for application of pressure might be available. With the woman in a high Fowler's position with a rounded back, a small, oblong sandbag can be placed behind the coccyx to support the lower back area. Other innovative ways to achieve the same type of pressure involve using two tennis balls (in socks to keep them from bouncing around), a rolling pin wrapped in a towel (especially a Tupperware rolling pin, which can be filled with hot or cold water to supply warmth or cold), or, in the absence of these, a firmly rolled towel.

Controlled Relaxation

Controlled relaxation is the foundation for all the respiratory techniques in labor. It becomes especially crucial in a back labor because tension in the lower back is particularly difficult to identify and release. Teaching controlled relaxation in the lateral position right at the beginning of the class series helps prepare the couple for this possibility. Stroking can signal relaxation, but it may be necessary for the labor coach to intone a reminder as well during active back labor contractions ("Relax your shoulders, back, buttocks, thighs," over and over). Evoking a sensual awareness by using terms like "Let your body feel warm and *melt* into the bed," "Let the tension *flow* out as you feel my hand," may be helpful. The woman may be encouraged to switch the focus of her concentration from her respiratory technique to active controlled release of tension from all the involved musculature.

Temperature

The fourth major possibility for increasing comfort is temperature. Heat is usually the most comforting, but a few women prefer the application of cold. At home a heating pad, hot water bottle, or ice bag may be used. In the hospital it depends upon what is available. A washcloth or towel could be applied to the area of discomfort as a hot or cold compress. An examination glove filled with ice chips and closed off with a rubber band is another possibility. If the couple chooses to use cold, they must be cautioned to protect the area against tissue damage by wrapping the ice-filled object with a towel before applying it directly to the skin.

Variation in the Progress of Labor

To simplify, problem labors can be categorized into roughly three types: problems with the passage, with the passenger, or with the powers of labor.

Passage

Problems with the passage include pelvic **contractures** (inlet, mid-pelvis, or outlet). If the contracture is in the pelvic inlet, the presentation may be altered because the presenting part cannot engage. The membranes may rupture and caput succedaneum forms early, but the presenting part cannot move down within the pelvis. Cephalopelvic disproportion must be suspected whenever the presenting part does not engage or does not descend within the pelvis as labor progresses.

Another anomaly of the passageway is cervical rigidity. When this occurs, there is usually a history of abortion, **conization**, or other surgery. The cervix effaces but fails to dilate. Hellman and Pritchard state that this is rarely the primary cause of **dystocia** and may usually be treated by augmentation of previously ineffective contractions.[9]

Very rarely, a constricted ring forms in the uterus, impeding further descent. In the past this was usually associated with protracted rupture of membranes and a long or obstructed labor. Clearer parameters dividing normal from prolonged labors as well as x-ray delineation of obstruction has practically eliminated this difficulty. Occasionally, a ringlike constriction forms following the birth of a first twin, but the use of deep general or epidural anesthesia usually relaxes it.[9]

Problems with the Passenger

By far the most common problem with the passenger is excessive size in relation to the mother's pelvis. This may be due to hereditary factors, such as a large father and a small mother, or to maternal diabetes. Some fetal anomalies also cause difficulty, such as the hydrocephalic whose head is too distended to engage or the anencephalic whose lack of a cranium is a poor dilating force against the cervix.

Malpositions or **malpresentations** cause further difficulty in fetal negotiation of the bony pelvis. If the fetal head is poorly flexed or is extended, as in a brow or face presentation, the broadest diameters of the fetal head must pass through the pelvis. This will take a prolonged time as a great deal of moulding must take place. The parents should be prepared for the fact that the infant's face will appear swollen and bruised because it has undergone considerable trauma. If the infant is at term, it is likely that a cesarean birth will be necessary.

The infant in a transverse lie has the shoulder presenting. This may happen if the mother has a pelvic contracture, if she has had many previous babies, or if a **placenta previa** obstructs the descent of the presenting part. If a transverse lie is found proir to the onset of labor, a cesarean birth will be scheduled because the labor contractions could result in uteroplacental insufficiency or in uterine rupture.

If the infant is in a breech position, the parents may be informed of this ahead of time and will ask how a breech birth differs from the usual birth. Certainly there is an increased risk. Because the fetus must dilate the cervix and pass through the birth canal using the smaller, softer body parts as a wedge, it takes longer. **Pelvimetry** must be done to be certain that the head can pass through the maternal bony structures. Because of the increased stress on the infant, a fetal monitor is used if available. There is an increased possibility of early rupture of membranes and, because the **presenting part** does not completely fill the pelvis, a risk of prolapsed cord. The parents should be prepared for the possiblity of cesarean birth.

The instructor must bear in mind that the malpresentation is freqently caused by other obstructive factors that prevent normal engagement and descent, such as placenta previa or constriction of the pelvis.

Powers of Labor

Dysfunctional or prolonged labor may be defined as a latent phase of more than 20 hours for primigravidas or 14 hours for multigravidas. Prolongation of the active phase is defined as progressive cervical dilatation of less than 1.2 cm/hour in primiparas and less than 1.5 cm/hour in multiparas.[9] Although these parameters must be applied individually, they do provide guidelines on which to assess the progress of labor and delineate the normal from the abnormal fairly promptly. The powers, of course, refer to the contractions. Dysfunctional contractions may be categorized as **hypotonic** or **hypertonic**, either of which may be responsible for prolongation of labor.

Hypertonic contractions usually occur in a prolonged latent phase and may be referred to as **primary uterine inertia**. These contractions are usually far more painful subjectively than can be accounted for by objective measurements. Although the pressure gradient is strong, hypertonic contractions may be distorted. For example, instead of originating in the fundus and exerting force downward against the passively contracting lower uterine segment, the contraction may be more forceful in the midsection than the fundus. Sometimes the contraction never becomes completely coordinated.

Fetal distress is common, perhaps because of interference with uteroplacental circulation. Cephalopelvic disproportion or mechanical obstruction must be considered.

Hypertonic dysfunction responds poorly to oxytocics. The treatment of choice is to sedate the mother to allow her to rest, either with parenteral medication or with epidural anesthesia. After the rest period, the woman usually goes into normal labor. If not, a mild trial of oxytocin may be tried. In the few cases in which sedation fails to stop the contractions, or in which the fetus is in distress, a cesarean birth may be necessary.

When the contractions are hypotonic, they do not exert enough force to effect the progressive changes in the cervix characteristic of normal labor. The fundus can be indented, even during the peak of the contraction. Hypotonic contractions may be caused by uterine or maternal exhaustion, by overmedication before true labor is well established, by mild pelvic contracture, or by fetal malposition.

Hypotonic dysfunction occurs in the active phase of labor when the cervix is at least 3 cm dilated and may be referred to as **secondary inertia**.

Fetal distress usually does not appear unless infection is present.

The woman may be given oxytocin after a vaginal exam and perhaps a pelvimetry has ruled out disproportion. The hypotonic type of contraction usually responds well to stimulation by oxytocin.

Precipitate Labor

Precipitate labor is defined as a labor lasting 3 hours or less. This is more common in multiparas. It may occur because the woman does not realize she is in labor until she is ready to deliver. It may be the result of very low resistance of the maternal soft parts as in the **grand multipara**, or it may be caused by excessively long and strong contractions, sometimes the result of oxytocics. In any case, the child is precipitated through the birth canal with little chance for accomodation of the fetal head. These babies often exhibit extreme moulding and may sustain cerebral trauma. Excessively long contractions interfere with uteroplacental exchange and may cause **anoxia**. An additional danger is the fact that precipitate delivery may take place without adequate arrangements for the infant in the crucial first minutes of life. If the woman has a history of precipitate delivery, her physician will probably consider an induction if conditions are favorable.

Induction or Stimulation of Labor

Indications

The couples who come to class may have heard about induction of labor or "babies by appointment" and wonder about this practice. The popularity of appointment babies has declined somewhat since the widespread use of fetal monitoring has underlined the additional stress to the fetus. There are medical indications for induction of labor, however. They include premature rupture of the membranes, a mother who is toxemic, diabetic, or hypertensive, or prolonged pregnancy with a falling estriol level—in short, any indication that the continuance of the pregnancy would be more hazardous to the fetus than the induction of labor.

Conditions must be favorable for the induced contractions to effect cervical change. To ascertain if the woman is a good candidate for induction, the physician evaluates certain criteria according to the **Bishop scale** (Table 7-1).

Application

There are several modes of inducing labor: **aminotomy**; sublingual, intranasal, or intravenous oxytocin; and most recently **prostaglandin**. The childbirth educator should be acquainted with the modes that are being used in her community so that she can prepare her students.

Oxytocin in either the sublingual or intranasal form is still employed in some parts of the United States. This can be an effective way to induce labor, but difficulty in controlling the length and strength of the contractions has sometimes led to dangerous tetanic contractions.

Amniotomy alone does not guarantee that labor will follow, committing the physician to delivery by cesarean section if the woman does not progress to the second stage within 24 hours. Amniotomy is often used in conjunction with oxytocin after good labor has been established and the presenting part is well engaged. Some feel that this practice is not without serious hazard to the fetus, however.[4]

Prostaglandins are produced by the uterus itself and are found in semen as well (see Sexual Activitiy Controversy and Concern, Chap. 5). For years, research into its action was hampered because the supply was dependent upon a biosynthetic process requiring seminal vesicles from

Table 7-1. **Bishop Scale for Determining Readiness for Induction of Labor**

Criteria evaluated	0 points	3 points
Cervical dilatation	0 cm	3 cm
Consistency of cervix	Firm	Soft
Cervical effacement	None	80%
Position of cervix	Posterior	Forward or central
Station of presenting part	−3	+2

The parturient is rated 0-3 on each of the criteria. A total score of less than 9 indicates a poor candidate for induction.

hundreds of thousands of sheep. The unexpected finding of prostaglandins in a type of coral found in the Caribbean Sea has relieved the supply problem, allowing for total synthesis.

Recently, the prostaglandins have been studied as possible alternatives to oxytocin. The studies have generally shown the prostaglandins to be at least as effective in inducing labor as the oxytocics used. However, the prostaglandins were slightly less predictable, producing an occasional tetanic contraction without warning, as well as frequent gastrointestinal side-effects. Presumably, experience over a period of time will result in more precise application and an improved therapeutic index. In all studies, the success rate correlated more closely with the Bishop scale scores than with the method of induction used.[2,6]

Most frequently, labor is induced by the use of intravenous oxytocin. This preparation may be either the natural preparation (Pitocin) or a synthetic analogue (Syntocinon). There are no remarkable differences in the oxytocic effects.[5] The advantage of this mode is that contractions can be regulated easily by either speeding or slowing the rate of infusion. In the event of hypertonus, the medication can be immediately terminated.

Commonly, a dose of between 3 and 10 units of oxytocin is mixed into a bottle of 500 or 1000 cc Ringer's lactate. This bottle of medicated solution is attached by a ϑ tube, or piggyback to the tubing of an already started infusion. The rate of medicated flow can be calibrated precisely by the use of an infusion pump. If necessary, the medication can be discontinued while the vein is kept open with fluid from the unmedicated bottle.

Sometimes labor must be induced before the cervix is fully ripe for example; if the membranes rupture prematurely. In this case the processes that normally occur over a period of weeks must take place in the space of a few hours. The woman may be admitted to the hospital and given up to 12 hours of oxytocin-induced contractions. Then the medication is discontinued, and she is allowed to rest for at least 8 hours. During the rest period the uterus may continue to contract (painlessly) so the cervix continues to ripen. It may be necessary to repeat this ripening process several times before the cervix is ready and adequate labor is established.

It is extremely important for the health care team to give the parents emotional support thoughtout this period. The idea of a "failed" induction extracts a heavy psychological toll. Adequate explanation emphasizing the preparation of the cervix rather than immediate progress helps.

Because there is an increased risk of postpartum hemorrhage when oxytocin is discontinued, usually the medication is continued until the completion of the bottle.[5]

Many hospitals mandate that the physician be physically present at all times while an induction is going on so that immediate intervention can be instituted if necessary. If available, the fetal monitor is also attached because of the increased stress on the infant.

Oxytocins may also be used to stimulate the labor if contractions become ineffective. In the absence of cephalopelvic disproportion or placental insufficiency, this is the treatment of choice for secondary inertia. It may also be necessary to stimulate labor if medication or extradural anesthesia is used too liberally or too early in labor.

Intramuscular oxytocin (sparteine sulfate) may also be used occasionally to stimulate labor. Because reactions vary and the dose cannot be reduced or withdrawn once the injection is given, extreme care must be observed.

The Mother's Reaction

The mother needs to know how labor induced or stimulated by oxytocin will feel to her and how it differs from the usual pattern. One change is in the character of the contractions. Induced contractions are of greater intensity and have shorter intervals. These contractions peak rapidly, necessitating a quicker entry into respiratory techniques, that is the first deep signal breath must proceed at a more rapid pace than would be necessary for a contraction with a longer increment. Because labor may progress more rapidly, the use of rhythmic chest breathing or modified rhythmic chest breathing may be minimal. (Breathing patterns are described in Appendix A.) The woman should be encouraged to advance to the combined or even shallow breathing if necessary to maintain control. She needs active coaching and may need to augment her technique with analgesia. She also should be informed that, although the labor is more intense than unaugmented labor, it is generally shorter.

Second Stage

Episiotomy

The most common of all obstetric operations, episiotomy is an incision into the perineum to enlarge the vaginal outlet. It is done to avoid possible overstretching or tearing of the perineum as well as to shorten the second stage and reduce trauma to the fetal head. While many obstetricians would agree with a mother's request to wait and see if an episiotomy is necessary, most find that the degree of stretching of the perineum is such that they ultimately decide in favor of episiotomy.

The incision is made either mediolaterally or midline, usually after an injection of local anesthetic, when the presenting part shows about 2 to 3 cm. The mother is only minimally aware of the procedure, because the pressure of the presenting part against local nerve endings as well as the impairment of circulation has a numbing effect on the perineum.

After the third stage is complete, the episiotomy is sutured with either absorbable chromic gut or with a polyglycolic acid (PGA) suture. The latter has been found by some to excite less tissue reaction than the traditional catgut and hence causes less episiotomy pain.[15]

The mother should resume her perineal contraction exercises immediately, even before the effects of local anesthetic have worn off, and do them every hour when awake (see Appendix A). Scrupulous perineal care, sitz baths, and heat lamp (or ice pack) can also reduce postpartum pain. Postpartum nursing care includes inspection for erythema, edema, and **hematoma**.

Forceps

Obstetric forceps are used to assist the delivery of the head or to rotate it to a more favorable position. Since expectant parents have many misconceptions about obstetric forceps, it is worthwhile to discuss the reasons for forceps delivery. Nonthreatening pictures of forceps and therapeutic words used in descriptions are helpful; for example, the instrument can be described as similar to salad tongs rather than blades.

When the cervix is fully dilated and the child moves down into the birth canal, forceps may be applied if it is deemed desirable to shorten the second stage. Fetal indications include fetal distress, umbilical cord **prolapse**, and malposition. Other indications might be an exhausted mother who is unable to sustain the pushing effort, ineffective contractions, premature separation of the placenta, or toxemia or cardiac disease in the mother.

The mother should know how and when forceps are applied. Low forceps (outlet forceps), which are the most frequently used, are applied when the head is already on the perineum, usually after injection of a pudendal nerve block or other regional anesthetic. Mid forceps are less frequently applied but may be helpful if a rotation is desirable and the mother's pushing efforts are ineffective. They would be used to rotate the fetus from a persistent occiput posterior or deep transverse arrest or to hasten delivery in cases of fetal distress.

High forceps have no place in the practice of modern obstetrics. Before advances in anesthesia and antibiotic therapy made cesarean birth a safe operation, high forceps were applied when the infant was still above the level of the ischial spines. This procedure was traumatic to both the fetus and mother; it sometimes resulted in palsies of the facial or brachial nerves or fractures of the clavicle for the fetus and in vaginal tears for the mother. Today a cesarean birth would be performed because it is less stressful to mother and fetus.

Birth reports indicate that low forceps application is not too uncomfortable for the parturient as long as adequate explanation is made. The mother must remain still and should be coached to use her controlled relaxation while the forceps are being applied. She may find it difficult to push down and at the same time hold back from being (as it feels to her) pulled toward the physician as he exerts force on the forceps.

Rare complications include a facial palsy or cephalhematoma, both transient, or maternal vaginal or perineal tears. Occasionally, trauma to the urethral meatus causes postpartum difficulty in voiding.

Cesarean Births

Thirteen percent of childbearing couples can expect to have a primary cesarean section, making preparation for cesarean delivery an important part of childbirth preparation. The amount of time devoted should reflect at least this percentage of total class time. Topics for discussion are included in more detail in Chapter 8; however, it is worthwhile mentioning cesarean birth briefly here to keep it within the general perspective of holistic preparation for variations of labor and delivery.

The first task will be to make the possibility of cesarean birth real. Couples tend to deny the possibility that a cesarean delivery could happen to them, and to selectively "tune out" this important topic. Awareness of this tendency will help the instructor create ways to help couples work out their coping options should this unwanted outcome occur. We know that the more actively couples can participate in their own learning, the more integrated that learning will be. Stimulating active discussion of what they have heard and believe can help meet this goal.

The instructor should begin by relating the indications for cesarean birth. The media has increased general awareness of cesarean birth but in some instances has left expectant parents with the idea that it is an evil against which they must be one their guard. This negative attitude burdens them and makes it difficult for them to be open to nonjudgmental data on indications for the cesarean choice. Emphasizing the couple's part in the decision-making process and the requirement of informed consent and signed release forms may help them to relax and listen.

Relating the discussion of indications for cesarean birth to previous discussions of available tests for fetal well-being will build on prior knowledge. The commonest indication for a primary cesarean section is cephalopelvic disproportion, followed by uterine inertia, placenta previa, and malposition or malpresentation. Other indications are toxemia, fetal distress, prolapsed cord, premature rupture of membranes, and active herpes genitalis.

The inclusion of posters depicting the delivery itself as well as giving a general outline of procedures followed will help build correct expectations. A movie or slide presentation to reinforce information would be invaluable. If this is beyond the reach of the instructor in private practice, she should consider the possibility of sharing resources, either with other instructors or by sending her students to a local hospital or childbirth education group film or slide show.

Preoperative Preparation

A cesarean may be performed with epidural anesthesia, with spinal anesthesia, or under general anesthesia. The major medical indication for a general anesthetic is the speed with which it can be used; if the fetus is in distress, this may be crucial. Usually a spinal or epidural anesthetic is possible, however. Then, if she wishes, the mother can remain awake to see and hear her child at the first possible moment.

A catheter is inserted preoperatively and remains in place to avoid bladder distention. The abdominal and pubic hair is shaved and the area washed with a cleansing solution. The mother receives an injection to dry up nasal secretions and an infusion is started. On the delivery table, a screen is placed at the level of the mother's shoulders so that she cannot directly observe the incision. If she wishes, the anesthetist, seated near her head monitoring her responses, may give her a running commentary. If the father is present to share the birth, he too is seated near her head and screened from watching the surgery.

Operation

The incision may be either a vertical or transverse "bikini" incision. After the incision is made into the uterus, the membranes are ruptured and the amniotic fluid suctioned. The infant is grasped and delivered manually or with forceps. The mother should be prepared to feel the sensation of tissue manipulation, even though she feels no pain; this heralds the birth of the baby, which may be as soon as 5 min after the surgery begins. The suturing and repair take about another 45 min.

The father, if he is present, should give the mother a description of all that is being done with and for the baby until she can see for herself. The nose and mouth are aspirated to assure a patent airway; the cord is clamped and cut. The child is then examined briefly, dried, and wrapped to prevent chilling. Then the father can show the baby to its mother.

If the father is not present, word should be sent to him as soon as the baby is born. A suggestion has been made that a Polaroid picture of the infant be taken if the mother has general anesthesia or if the father is not present. This helps to make the transition from pregnancy to parenting more real.[1]

Postoperative Care

In most hospitals the mother is taken to the recovery room where she remains until she has recovered from the anesthetic and her vital signs have stabilized. Because of the critical nature of the first hour for maternal–infant bonding, some hospitals allow the infant to remain with her in recovery. The father and mother together can get acquainted with their new child.

The infusion is usually continued overnight, and the catheter remains in place for a day or so. The mother is usually restricted to a liquid diet until bowel sounds are heard or until she begins to pass gas.

The incision will be sore. The mother should be encouraged to use medication for pain if she needs it, for this will help her feel more able to handle her baby. She should be encouraged to get out of bed and begin walking within 12 to 18 hours. She can be shown how to splint the incision with both hands for support and (see Fig. 8–1) and should be urged to gently contract and release the abdominal muscles. This helps to avoid muscle stiffness and improves her ability to pass intestinal gas. She should do this maneuver five times every hour when awake.

The mother who has had a cesarean birth can breastfeed just as successfully as any other new mother. The major difficulty lies in her inability to move around and handle her child easily. She can be encouraged to nurse either in the side-lying position or with a pillow over her abdomen to prevent pain caused by pressure from the infant's weight.

Because of the increased blood supply to the uterus during and immediately following pregnancy, healing is rapid. The mother may be discharged after 5 to 8 days, when the stitches are removed. However, the family needs to see that she has adequate help when she first goes home.

Emotional Recovery

Because the emotional impact of birth can influence postpartum adjustments, it is worthwhile exploring the special needs of the woman who delivers her child by cesarean. Although she may express relief, especially if the surgery followed a long and arduous labor or if there was fetal distress, it is always tinged with regret that the birth experience was not what the couple had worked and planned for together. The woman may feel that she has failed in the ultimate feminine function of giving birth. This will surely affect her self-esteem and confidence in herself as a mother. Although she may deny it, she may feel slightly hostile toward the baby or toward its father for being the cause of her pain. These negative feelings may be around for a long time and color the new parenting role.

Childbirth teachers do not like emphasizing problems in class; they always try to give confidence by stressing the positive. Some couples interpret this to mean that discipline in practice and application of technique will avert any and all problems. The possibility of problems may be denied: "It won't happen to me." Cesarean birth should be mentioned in early classes as an alternative mode of delivery, *not* saved for the class about delivery as if it were a major catastrophe. The instructor can help the couples to think about possible alternatives and dispel some of the myths surrounding cesarean birth. Emotional support comes from keeping the emphasis on the *birth* aspect rather than on the surgery. The infant is not a side benefit of the operation; this is a new member of a family, whatever mode of birth is necessary. The new mother has all the needs of a postoperative patient, but she experiences all the needs of a new mother as well.

Postpartum, the need to verbalize feelings about a cesarean birth are even more crucial than with a vaginal birth. The mother needs to be reassured that nothing she did or could have done could have changed the outcome. She is not to blame. The "never mind, be glad you have a healthy infant" approach is not helpful, because it fails to recognize the mother's feelings of sadness.

Third Stage

Lacerations

Sometimes lacerations occur in the cervix, vagina, or perineum, especially if the delivery is precipitate, if the infant is large, or if forceps were applied.

Perineal lacerations or extensions of the episiotomy include first-degree lacerations (involving only the fourchette and skin of the perineum and vaginal mucosa), second-degree lacerations (involving the skin, mucous membrane, and muscle layers of the perineum), and third-degree lacerations (which include all of the above and extend into the anal sphincter). Occasionally, third-degree lacerations also involve the anterior wall of the rectum. The more serious tears require careful approximation of each of the layers. Postpartum complications include pain, difficulty in voiding or defecation, and occasional hematoma. The comfort measures are the same as for episiotomy, and the mother should practice her perineal contraction exercise gently, but faithfully.

Retained Placenta

Retained placenta is a rather rare complication. The parents need to be prepared for this eventuality because a simple explanation ahead of time can keep it from being magnified in their minds to major proporations. If the obstetrician finds that the placenta is not whole, the remainder must be manually removed. Although this is uncomfortable for the mother, a regional anesthetic or momentary general anesthetic usually suffices. She will awaken within minutes and, hopefully, the baby and labor coach will still be there. If she remains awake, she can return to her controlled relaxation and shallow breathing.

This usually takes place before the episiotomy repair.

Hemorrhage

One of the most serious of the postpartum complications is hemorrhage. It can be caused by laceration, retained placenta fragments, or uterine **atony**. An oxytocic is usually given following the third stage to prevent uterine relaxation.

In the immediate **puerperium** the fundus looks to the mother rather like a small grapefruit halfway between the symphysis and the umbilicus. The nurse may massage it or teach the mother to do so to stimulate contraction to compress the placental site. The mother can be told to expect bleeding similar to menstrual bleeding (*i.e.*, no large clots) but to report uterine relaxation (a soft, boggy feeling), large clots, or large amounts of fresh bleeding to the nurse.

Occasionally postpartum hemorrhage occurs after the first 24 hours, but before the end of the first month. This is usually due to retained placental fragments or **subinvolution** of the placental site. The treatment is immediate hospitalization and dilation and curettage (**D and C**) to remove the placental fragments.

Preparing the High-Risk Mother

Pregnancy and childbirth are normally stressful, involving changes in relationships and family roles. If the outcome of the pregnancy is in doubt, the stress is intensified and exacts a heavy toll on the parents' psychological reserves.

The expectant mother who is struggling with the task of adapting her self-image from "who she is" to "who she will become" is also experiencing changes in her body image from "not pregnant" to "full of life." If she is high risk as well, the "pregnant" image may become "defective carrier." The result can be disastrous to her self-esteem. The woman may fear not only for her child and for herself, but also for her relationship with the baby's father. She may fear rejection because she sees herself as failing in the womanly function of childbearing. Her fears about the outcome of the pregnancy interfere with her ability to form an internalized image of her infant as an intact human being and may contribute to maladaptive behavior toward the pregnancy or toward the infant.

A grieving process takes place, characterized by the following:

Denial. "I feel well; how can there be anything wrong?" "It can't be happening to me."

Anger and Guilt. "Why me?" If only I had (stuck to my diet, not taken those pills)." "Maybe this is our punishment because we didn't want this pregnancy in the beginning."

Plea Bargaining and Magical Thinking. "If only everything turns out all right I'll never. . . ."

Acceptance. Finally, in the healthy couple, some acceptance of the pregnancy as it is.

The marriage may come under great stress at this time unless the couple can discuss their mutual needs and feelings. The nurse or childbirth educator who may be counseling the couple can help them to support each other by stressing the importance of good communication. If the couple can learn to nurture each other in such times of stress, their bond will be strengthened.

Communication is especially important between all members of the childbirth team to provide support and continuity of care for the high-risk family. A great number of tests must be done to monitor the well-being of the fetus and the efficiency of the uteroplacental unit, and they are expensive in terms of time, trouble, and money. Maternal health care providers can influence the family's ability to accept and adapt by giving adequate explanations and providing time for both parents to ventilate their feelings. Each test must be explained and the results interpreted for them. The more they can be included in planning their own care, the less helpless they will feel.

In addition to listening empathetically, the educator can help them to mobilize their coping mechanisms by asking judicious questions such as "What will you do?", "What plans have you made?" and by making appropriate referrals.[7]

Those women who fall into the high-risk category can be identified on the basis of statistical studies of fetal mortality and morbidity. They include

1. Women with a poor obstetric history (history of stillbirth, prematurity, or abnormality)
2. Grand multiparas (five or more pregnancies)
3. Chronic users of hard drugs
4. Women with Rh incompatability (previous pregnancy, abortion, or miscarriage not treated with RhoGAM)
5. Chronically ill women (diabetics other than Class A, hypertensives)
6. Women under 16 or over 35 years of age
7. Nutritionally deprived women

Diagnostic Tests

Amniocentesis

Amniocentesis is the withdrawal of 10 to 20 cc amniotic fluid under sterile conditions by means of a needle through the abdominal wall into the amniotic sac. Prior to the procedure sonography is done to locate the placenta. The woman is then instructed to empty her bladder. The fetus is palpated to identify the optimal site for insertion of the needle. The fetal heart tones are recorded (rechecked following the procedure and every 15 min for 1 hour afterwards), or the mother is placed on the external fetal monitor.

The skin is cleansed, the needle inserted, and the fluid withdrawn.

There is often an increase in uterine activity for a short while following the procedure, but this generally returns to normal within the hour.

There have been reports of the fetus being punctured, maternal hemorrhage, or infection following the procedure, but the incidence is less than 1%.[12]

Amniocentesis can provide information about genetic disorders (such as Down's syndrome), hereditary metabolic disorders (such as Tay-Sachs), and sex-linked defects (such as hemophilia). These conditions are diagnosed by cell cultures grown from the amniotic fluid. Because each disorder must be cultured for specifically, which is time consuming and expensive, there must be adequate justification for each test, such as a family history of the disorder. Since amniocentesis can be performed in early pregnancy, the parents may choose to interrupt the pregnancy if a disorder is found rather than bear an afflicted child. By means of amniocentesis they may also be reassured when the fetus is *not* a victim of a familial disorder. Amniocentesis can also identify the sex of the fetus through chromosomal studies.

In the last trimester, amniocentesis may be performed to assess the maturity of the fetal lungs by a lecithin-**sphingomyelin** (L–S) ratio. Prior to 35 weeks gestation, the amounts of the phospholipids lecithin and sphingomyelin in a 5-cc sample of amniotic fluid remain fairly constant. At 35 to 36 weeks, the fetal alveolar cells begin to produce **surfactant,** the main component of which is **lecithin.** Surfactant reduces the surface tension in the alveoli and maintains their stability so that they do not collapse on expiration. When progressive collapse of the respiratory lobule does occur, it contributes to **respiratory distress syndrome (RDS).**[16]

Because of intrauterine fetal respiratory movements in late pregnancy, lecithin begins to flow into the surrounding amniotic fluid, and the lecithin–to–sphingomyelin ratio begins to increase. If the L–S ratio is 1.5:1 or less, the lung is immature and the risk of the newborn developing RDS is quite high. If L:S has increased to 2:1 or more, RDS is rarely seen.[16]

Estriol Measurement

The placenta converts steroid precursors produced by the fetal adrenals into the estrogen product estriol. Hence, adequate or high levels of estriol in maternal serum or urine reflect a well-integrated and active fetoplacental unit.[16] The values increase throughout pregnancy until at term, 24-hour (urine) values may vary 12 to 50 mg/24 hours. Because the measurements can vary from day to day, single measurements are of little value and serial tests are usually performed. The patient must bring in a 24-hour urine specimen, preferably on consecutive or alternate days. If the mother is considered to be at risk, long intervals are contraindicated.

Sometimes a serum **estriol** test is done either in conjunction with or instead of a urinary estriol test. The serum estriol measurement reflects immediate levels, whereas the 24-hour urine specimen reflects functional efficiency for the previous 24 hours.

The urinary estriol test is less reliable if there is any malfunctioning of the mother's liver or kidney that might interfere with conjugation or excretion. In the case of a low estriol level a creatinine clearance test may be done to check for renal function. If both values are decreased, renal disease may be suspected.[11]

Other conditions that may interfere with accurate estriol values include a less-than-complete 24-hour specimen; severe anemia; and maternal intake of ampicillin, steroids, stool softeners such as Agoral, Evac-Q Kit, Prulet, phenolphthalein (Sarolax) or methenamine mandelate (Mandelamine).

Concentrations of less than 7 mg/24 hours or a drop of more than 25% from the patient's previous test may indicate that the fetus is in jeopardy. A value of less than 3 mg/24 hours usually indicates fetal death.[7,11]

There are no hazzards to the mother or fetus in estriol testing. Burosh has suggested that the three criteria that should be followed for effective use of estriol testing are

1. More than one serial determination
2. No long intervals between tests
3. No intervention on the basis of only one borderline value[3]

Indications for ordering estriol determinations include toxemia, post datism and intrauterine growth retardation.

One of the major values of estriol testing is that it shows whether the fetus is in immediate danger or whether it may safely remain *in utero* for a while longer. This may be crucial if there is an element of increasing risk, and the obstetrician must decide when to intervene.

Ultrasound

Ultrasound testing is done by sending low-intensity sound waves through the patient's body. The waves are reflected back at tissue interfaces, and are received by the **transducer** and translated onto an **oscilloscope** as a "picture" made up of electrical blips. Ultrasound in pregnancy can reveal important information about gestational age, fetal head growth, placental site (important prior to amniocentesis, cesarean birth, or in cases where placenta previa is suspected), multiple pregnancies, and some abnormalities such as hydatid mole and anencephaly.

The **biparietal** diameter is measured to ascertain gestational age and, serially, to measure growth in head size. Although the biparietal diameter differs somewhat from fetus to fetus, parameters have been derived from data obtained by measuring fetuses of women who were certain of the date of their last menstrual periods. The dates were later confirmed by course of pregnancy and onset of labor. From this data a normal curve correlating gestational age with biparietal measurements was plotted.[7]

If intrauterine growth retardation is suspected, ultrasound testing may be repeated at 2-week intervals to determine if there has been an appropriate increase in fetal head size.

The mother is instructed to arrive for testing with a full bladder, because a full bladder displaces the uterus upward and seems to allow for a better scan. She is placed on the examination table, mineral oil is applied to her abdomen to increase conductivity, and the ultrasound transducer is passed over her abdomen.[7] The mother can watch the small screen and can see the picture forming from the electrical blips. The technician may point out the fetal outlines and often gives her a picture to keep. Many pregnant women who have been given copies of the ultrasound scans carry them around as if reassured of the continued good health of the fetus.

The procedure takes about 15–60 min, depending on fetal activity and position. To date, no adverse effects have been reported.[16]

Oxytocin Challenge Test

In cases of suspected placental insufficiency, an oxytocin challenge test (OCT), or stress test, may be done. It is well known that the exchange of gases and circulation is impaired during uterine contractions. If the respiratory function of the placenta is decreased before labor begins, the added stress of labor on an already compromised exchange places the fetus in increased danger of hypoxia or **acidosis.**

It may take up to 3 hours to obtain an adequate tracing. The mother comes in for her OCT, empties her bladder, and puts on a hospital gown. She is placed in a semirecumbent position or on her left side to reduce pressure on the inferior vena cava. Two transducers from the external fetal monitor are applied to record fetal heart rate and uterine contractions. The transducers, each about the size of a cigarette pack, are placed on the mother's abdomen and held in place by elastic straps.

A baseline recording is made of the fetal heart rate before the intravenous oxytocin is started. The rate of the oxytocin drip is gradually increased until the contractions are adequate. The mother's blood pressure is recorded every 10 min throughout the test.

A positive test, indicating inadequate uteroplacental reserves, results when there are late decelerations occurring during most contractions (see Fetal Monitoring). This is an indication that the fetus is endangered. Tests for fetal maturity are then carried out to ascertain how soon the baby may safely be delivered.

A negative OCT (no evidence of late decelerations) has been interpreted to mean that the fetus may safely remain *in utero* for at least 1 more week. If uteroplacental efficiency is in doubt (*e.g.*, for a toxemic or diabetic mother), OCTs should be repeated weekly to monitor placental efficiency until term.

Fetal Monitoring

Electronic fetal monitoring is becoming more prevalent for so-called normal as well as high-risk labors. Therefore, a discussion of fetal monitoring should be included in childbirth classes.

Indications

The fetal monitor measures the fetal heart rate (FHR) as well as the quality of uterine contractions. The tracing shows not only bradycardia (under 120 beats per minute) and **tachycardia** (over 160 beats per minute), which are variations in the baseline reading, but also variations of acceleration or deceleration that occur in relation to the contractions. This relationship is essential information for assessing problems.

The most common cause of perinatal morbidity (such as neurologically impaired or cerebral-palsied children) or mortality is **intrapartal** hypoxia. This may be caused in labor by interference with oxygen transport to the fetus during hypertonic contractions or by placental insufficiency or cord compression. In the healthy fetal–placental unit the oxygen reserves are such that the heart rate does not slow with contractions. When persistent decelerations do occur, it can be considered abnormal and the cause should be sought.[10]

Electronic monitoring has the advantage of maintaining a constant record of heart rate during and immediately following the contraction, which may be difficult to obtain through **auscultation.** If auscultation is delayed even 30 sec after the contraction, valuable information has been lost; any variability in rate may have disappeared by that time. Thus, the monitor is most valuable in detecting signs of fetal distress before they become so gross that they can be detected by intermittent auscultation alone. Only one study has disputed this.[8]

Admittedly, fetal monitoring is still in the early stages of refinement. When used in conjunction with acid–base evaluation of the fetus, however, it is the most accurate and objective measurement available for obstetric management.

Meaning of Tracings

The tracings make it possible to evaluate beat-to-beat variations as well as accelerations or decelerations in relation to the contractions. Normally there is some beat-to-beat variation, which increases with fetal movement or during the second stage of labor, perhaps as a result of increased tactile stimulation.[13] When beat-to-beat variability decreases, it is necessary to look for the cause. Drugs may effect variability either by central nervous system depression (barbiturates, tranquilizers, narcotics, anesthetics), by interfering with control impulses to the cardiac pacemaker (atropine, scopolamine), or by causing maternal hypotension, which interferes with uterine perfusion.[13] A more ominous reason for smoothing of the heart rate variability is central nervous system depression due to severe hypoxia and acidosis.

Some *acceleration* occurs with fetal movement, but this is not considered an ominous sign. If acceleration persistently occurs with contractions, it may be a sign of fetal compromise.

Decelerations in the fetal heart rate that occur early in the contraction (before the peak) are termed *early decelerations.* The mechanism is believed to be compression on the fetal head; the increased intracranial pressure interferes with circulation to the fetal brain (Fig. 7-2, *A*). Early decelerations are usually thought to be innocuous, although some would disagree.[4,10]

Late decelerations are thought to be caused by uteroplacental insufficiency and are a direct result of the decrease in intervillous flow (maternal–fetal exchange); hence, the decelerations occur late in the contraction (Fig. 7-2, *B*). They may be associated with uterine hypertonicity or hyperactivity or with maternal hypotension.

Late decelerations are an ominous sign and may be treated by treating the hyperactivity, changing the mother's position to relieve pressure on the inferior vena cava and aorta, administering oxygen, and correcting any hypotensive state.[10] The drop in variable deceleration rates is not temporally related to the contraction. *Variable decelerations* are thought to be the result of cord compression (Fig. 7-2, *C*), and a primary measure in treatment is to change the maternal position. Administration of oxygen has not been shown to be effective since the occlusion of the cord interferes with all placental–fetal exchange.[10] If the decelerations are persistent and fetal blood sampling indicates that the fetus is becoming acidotic, immediate steps must be taken to effect the birth.

External Monitoring

External monitoring can be used prior to labor or early in labor when the membranes are not ruptured and the cervix is not dilated. The fetal heartbeat may be detected either by amplification, as with phonocardiograms, or by the use of an ultrasonic transducer, which detects differences in frequency between the transmitted and reflected waves. In both methods the sound waves are amplified and recorded on a strip tape similar to the strip tape used in electrocardiograms.

The ultrasonic transducer is attached to the mother's abdomen by means of an elastic strap. Another elastic strap attaches a pressure sensitive

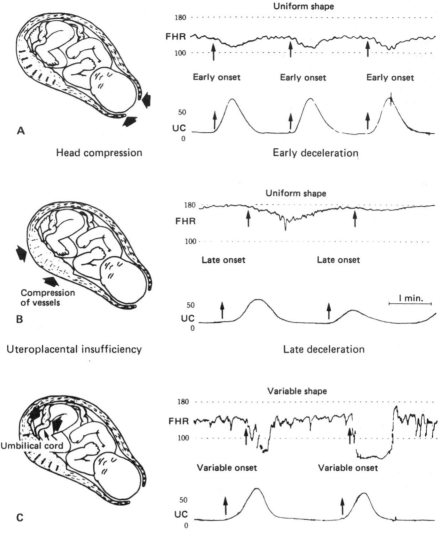

FIG. 7–2. (A) This FHR deceleration pattern is thought to be due to fetal head compression. It is of uniform shape, reflects the shape of the associated intrauterine pressure curve, and has its onset early in the contracting phase of the uterus. Hence, it has been labeled "early deceleration." UC=uterine contraction. (B) This FHR deceleration pattern is thought to be due to acute uteroplacental insufficiency as the result of decreased intervillous space blood flow during uterine contractions. It is also of uniform shape and also reflects the shape of the associated intrauterine pressure curve. In this case, however, in contradistinction to the uniform FHR deceleration pattern of A, its onset occurs late in the contracting phase of the uterus. Hence, it has been labeled "late deceleration." This FHR deceleration pattern is considered indicative of uteroplacental insufficiency. (C) This FHR pattern is thought to be due to umbilical cord occlusion. It is of variable shape and does not reflect the shape of the associated intrauterine pressure curve, and its onset occurs at a variable time during the contracting phase of the uterus. (Hon EH: An Introduction to Fetal Heart Rate Monitoring. Los Angeles, University of Southern California, 1973. Copyright by the author.)

transducer to the abdomen to measure the strength of the contraction. The advantage of the external monitor is that it is noninvasive and is not likely to cause infection or soft-tissue trauma.

Unfortunately, the external monitor produces inaccurate tracings when the mother moves, making frequent adjustments necessary. The mother may hesitate to assume a comfortable position because she dislikes "bothering" the labor room staff. Another disadvantage is that the supine position may be the best position for obtaining a clear reading. When this position results in supine hypotension and a late deceleration pattern, the patient may be turned on her side. Relieved that the monitor was able to discover the problem before it became too serious, she may not recognize the iatrogenic nature of the abnormality.

Internal Monitoring

After the membranes have ruptured and the cervix is dilated at least 2 cm, the internal or direct fetal monitor may be applied. First a Teflon, fluid-filled catheter is introduced into the uterus to measure the pressure gradient of the contraction. Following this a small spiral electrode is attached directly to the presenting part, with care to avoid the fontanelles.

The main advantage of direct monitoring is the increased accuracy due to diminished interference from maternal sounds. It also allows more freedom of movement for the mother. However, it requires rupture of the membranes, a practice that has been implicated in the increased incidence of head and cord compression because it removes the protective fluid cushion. Rare complications include fetal scalp infections, dislodging of the fetal head in order to introduce the uterine catheter, and uterine perforation.

Studies to date have failed to prove definitively that fetal outcome is improved with routine monitoring, although no one would argue the benefits accrued with monitoring the high-risk patient.

Meaning to Parents

Most childbirth instructors have viewed electronic monitoring for the low-risk patient with mixed emotions. On the one hand, monitoring has undoubtedly rescued many infants who have suffered from anoxia due to placental insufficiency or cord compression. On the other hand, it involves further instrumentation or intrusion into the already depersonalized birth process. The psychological impact of all the tubes and instrumentation upon parents is yet to be measured.

A word of caution should be interjected here. The instructor owes it to her students to present the pros and cons of monitoring without bias. It is mandatory for her to be aware of current practices in her own community so that she can prepare her students. The way in which this material is presented has a heavy impact upon patient acceptance and adaptation.

Monitoring can be presented as a helpful tool for the couple themselves to use, since the monitor can begin to register the contraction before it is perceptible to the mother. If the contractions are irregular or if the mother is fatigued and less aware of her contractions, the labor coach can use the monitor to give the verbal cue for institution of respiratory technique, as well as to let the mother know when the peak is over, that is, when she can expect the contraction to diminish in intensity.

References

1. Allan R: The caesarean birth experience. Presented at the Annual Symposium of Council of Childbirth Education Specialists, Inc., Tarrytown, New York, October 30, 1976
2. Anderson G, Hobbins J, Speroff L, Caldwell B: Intravenous prostaglandins E_2 and F_2 and Syntocinon for induction of term labor. J. Reprod Med 9:287-291, 1972
3. Burosh P: Serial estriol determinations in high risk pregnancies. JOGN Nurs 5(3):37, 1976
4. Caldeyro-Barcia R: Some consequences of obstetrical interference. Birth and the Family Journal 2:34-38, 1975
5. Fields H, Greene J, Smith K: Induction of Labor. New York, MacMillan, 1965
6. Friedman E, Sachtleben M, Green W: Oral prostaglandin E_2 for induction of labor at term. Am J Obstet Gynecol 123:667-674, 1975
7. Galloway K: Placental evaluation studies: The procedures, their purposes, and the nursing care involved. Matern Child Nurs J 1:300-306, 1976
8. Havercamp AD, Thompson HE, McFee JJ, Cetrulo C: The evaluation of continuous fetal heart rate monitoring in high risk pregnancy. Am J Obstet Gynecol 125:310, 1976
9. Hellman LM, Pritchard JA: Williams Obstetrics, 14th ed. New York, Appleton-Century-Crofts, 1971
10. Hon EH: An Introduction to Fetal Heart Rate Monitoring. Los Angeles, University of Southern California, 1973 (copyright by the author)
11. Jones M: Antepartum assessment in high risk pregnancy. JOGN Nurs 4(6):23-27, 1975
12. Korones S: High Risk Newborn Infants, St. Louis, CV Mosby, 1972
13. Martin C, Gingerich B: Factors affecting fetal heart rate. JOGN Nurs 5(Suppl):305-405, 1976
14. Nelson G, Byrans C: A comparison of oral prostaglandin E_2 and intravenous oxytocin for induction of labor in normal and high risk pregnancies. Am J Obstet Gynecol 126:549-554, 1976
15. Richardson A, Lyon J, Graham E, Williams N: Decreasing postpartum sexual abstinence time. Am J Obstet Gynecol 126:415-417, 1976
16. Status of the Fetus and Newborn. Columbus, OH, Ross Laboratories, 1973

8

Cesarean Birth Classes

With the increased cesarean rate and the general belief that women who have a uterine scar from previous surgery should not labor for a vaginal birth, the need for a class devoted to the special needs of the woman or couple who expect a cesarean delivery has arisen. Fully one third of all cesarean births are a result of previous cesarean delivery (about 7% of total births).

The rationale for preparation is the same as for couples who expect a vaginal birth. Well-thought-out physical and psychological preparation can play a major role in assisting couples to integrate the birth into their cycle of life events, showing respect for the social bonds of the new family unit, as well as diminishing some unwanted aftereffects of the surgery. Feelings of dissatisfaction surrounding cesarean birth most frequently focus on psychological events. Women complain of not being told what was going on, of fear because procedures were not understood, of isolation, of alienation, and of being disregarded as an adult participant in the birth drama. Studies of how people cope with stress indicate that the more control the person feels she has in a particular situation, the more ego enhancing it becomes in spite of setbacks. Protecting her sense of being in control as she necessarily loses control of her body processes is an important step in safeguarding her self esteem.[3] Some would argue that cesarean birth is solely the responsibility of the obstetrician, that the parents have no role because they cannot actively participate during the surgery. This is true to the extent that we are not advocating that the father assist the obstetrician, or that he cut the cord. However, working through the crisis of the birth is a process of adaptation for this expectant couple as well as for the couple attending the regular childbirth education class. Adaptation evolves out of reflexes and instincts, plus efforts to develop mastery through effective and well-practiced coping efforts. The instructor who believes that adaptation can be anticipatory as well as reactive, that people frequently approach anticipated stress with plans (taking on those that seem to have some possibility of being helpful, and seeking knowledge and feedback), can set the stage for new efforts in uncharted directions by offering learning, practice, and rehearsal in the cesarean birth class. By giving a realistic idea of what will occur, why it will occur, and what the mother or couple can do to enhance the process, the instructor assists the couple in building an expectation so that they can rehearse their response to it. She encourages communication and sometimes gives coaching in communication skills so that the couple can get their needs met. She gives information about the event and the reasons for the event, as well as variations and options available. She encourages couples to make decisions when they are appropriate, and to state their preferences. She informs them of their rights on controversial issues, and states the positive and the negative in a nonjudgemental way so that the couple will be able to make their own decisions. Personal preference of the instructor is identified as such. Table 8–1 outlines the possible structure for classes in cesarean birth preparation.

In the cesarean birth class the overwhelming majority of participants will have had a previous cesarean birth. Because of this, one of the major tasks of the initial session should be to open up discussion of the previous birth and to try to elicit unresolved negative feelings relating to it. The couple will not be ready to deal with the coming birth until questions and sad feelings about the past have been laid to rest. These angry feelings may have been difficult for the couple to identify and express at the time because of their relief at a positive outcome. With help, and in the safety of a group who have all experienced some negative feelings, they may be able to admit to and resolve these feelings.

This point is worth dwelling on. This mechanism of denial will frequently cause the first response to questioning to be, "It was OK; I was just happy that it was all over and that the baby was all right." The neutrality of this statement, that the birth drama was only "OK," should leave the instructor suspicious that there is a lot left unsaid that will cloud the person's ability to prepare for the coming birth; therefore, it is worth delving into. Because the overriding feeling was one of joy or relief does not exclude the human possibility of concurrent disappointment that the birth was not what the couple had hoped and planned for. At the time it may have seemed inappropriate to express doubts or questions about the birth. In trying to be supportive to new parents, too many of us have a tendency to gloss over the rough parts and stress the positive: "Well, at least it turned out well and the baby is all right." We need to recognize and empathize with legitimate feelings of anger and disappointment, and to prevent them from being bottled up and interfering with new parenting tasks.

In the first session the childbirth educator should spend enough time to allow each couple to talk about their previous experience, and to get to know the other class members somewhat. This presupposes a small group. The instructor is working to identify commonalities and to meld this collection of individuals into a working, mutually supportive group. Concurrently, the instructor is assessing the needs of this particular group. This is as much a part of the group work as the actual delivery of course materials, as every childbirth instructor knows.

After the initial interaction and mutal agreement on course objectives,

Table 8-1. Sample Class Outline for Cesarean Birth Preparation

Class	Content	Rationale
1	Introduce self, background; introduce local cesarean birth support group, if any.	To offer self as valid resource person; to reinforce need for resources for expectant and new cesarean parents
	Have students introduce themselves and state their goals. Discuss previous cesarean birth experiences.	To assess learner needs and to ventilate and clarify feelings
	Course overview	To assess needs of group (expectations and consensus)
	Discuss indications for cesarean birth.	To promote understanding, essential for active informed participation
	Discuss tests for fetal well-being and maturity.	To increase knowledge
	Discuss how physical conditioning prepares the body for stress of cesarean birth and recovery.	To provide motivation for practice
	Teach physical conditioning exercises.	To improve fitness, circulation, muscle tone; to promote high-level wellness
	Discuss nutrition, assessing students' own diets. Hand out dietary intake sheets.	To motivate, interest, and enlist participation
	Teach controlled relaxation (preparatory exercise only).	To create awareness of tension and relaxation; to promote rest, relaxation
2	Review previous class and answer questions.	To clarify, enlarge upon previous material
	Collect dietary intake sheets. Observe physical fitness exercises.	To reinforce, motivate
	Discuss hospital admission procedures, hospital tour, fetal maturity tests, p.r.n., signs of impending labor, preparation for surgery, anesthesiologist visit, choices.	To structure expectations, as anticipatory guidance
	Discuss the surgery, anesthesia administration, delivery room setup and procedures. Describe the surgery, procedure, sensations.	To promote realistic expectations
	Define coaching role. (Where does coach sit, what will he observe, when and under what conditions may he move around the room?)	To define coach's role, allay anxiety
	Discuss appearance of the baby, its needs, immediate postpartum care. Discuss recovery room: postpartum care of mother, pain medication, expectations, who will be present.	To promote realistic expectations
	Review controlled relaxation, slow rhythmic chest breathing.	To enhance comfort, control

(continued)

Table 8-1. **Sample Class Outline for Cesarean Birth Preparation**
(*continued*)

Class	Contents	Rationale
3	Review previous classes and answer questions. Observe all techniques.	To clarify, reinforce
	Overview recovery process, involution, foley, IV, nasogastric tube, postpartum pain, and medication.	To increase knowledge and provide correct expectations
	Demonstrate comfort positions for nursing/feeding. Teach exercises to enhance comfort: splinting abdomen, huffing, abdominal tightening, leg bracing, foot and ankle rotations, leg sliding, pelvic rocking, perineal contraction. Demonstrate turning in bed (side rails up, splint abdomen with pillows), getting out of bed.	To enhance comfort, promote circulation and healing
	Discuss diet and nutrition, their relationship to rapid healing (bran; no iced liquids or straws; no milk [may cause cramping, gas]; no gas-forming vegetables).	To provide anticipatory guidance, and to prevent discomfort
	Discuss prenatal vitamins (also postpartum vitamin C and iron when home).	To create awareness of nutritional needs
	Discuss extended postpartum diet, vitamins, rest, fluids, exercise. Discuss need for help at home, postpartum checkup, contraception.	To encourage planning
	Discuss preparing siblings (helping with feelings, sibling developmental tasks).	To provide anticipatory guidance
	Present slides or movie of cesarean birth, if available.	To promote realistic expectations, integration of knowledge
	Review controlled relaxation.	To reinforce need for rest, stress reduction
	Discuss need for cesarean support group.	To build resources for postpartum period, each other, self

the session moves into the content phase. Class content includes information that the couple need to give them a realistic expectation, thorough knowledge of the experience to come, and a feeling of preparedness that comes with understanding of options and procedures. They need to know why they needed to have the first cesarean, and why it is now anticipated that it will be repeated. They need to clarify this point to know that they are not to blame, either by act of omission or commission. Some in the class may be anticipating a possible vaginal delivery following a previous cesarean birth. They will need to be prepared for emergency cesarean delivery, but will need some guidance about what they can do to minimize the possibility or necessity of another cesarean birth. The International Childbirth Education Association has published a booklet entitled *Unnecessary Cesareans: Ways to Avoid Them,* which is available from the International Childbirth Education Association (ICEA) and may be suggested reading for class members.

Questions that cesarean couples can be encouraged to ask include the following:

1. Why is a cesarean birth necessary in my case?
2. Must I be admitted the day before the surgery? Or can I be admitted the morning of the surgery?
3. Will I have an IV and catheter? If so, for how long?
4. What area will be shaved?
5. Will my arms be strapped during the surgery? Will they be strapped at the wrist, or at the elbow so I can touch the baby?
6. Will there be a drape in place? Will there be a mirror so I can watch my child be born (if desired)?
7. What kind of incision will be made? What about my old scar?
8. Can the baby's father participate? What are the requirements?
9. What kind of anesthesia will be used?
10. Will the general operating room be used, or a delivery room?
11. Can baby and father be present in recovery? Can instillation of eyedrops be delayed?
12. Will the baby have to be in intensive care, or can the baby go to the regular nursery if his condition permits? If in ICN, for how long?
13. What if I have a fever?

These questions will help them to structure their ideas about the surgery and recovery period and to plan their coping strategies.[2]

Indications for Cesarean Birth

The most common indication for a cesarean birth is a uterine scar from a previous cesarean birth. Although the American College of Obstetricians and Gynecologists has released a statement that vaginal delivery after cesarean may be considered safe under proper conditions, many obstetricians still feel that once a woman has a scar on her uterus, subsequent births must always be by cesarean. Criteria for safe consideration of vaginal delivery following cesarean are discussed at the end of the chapter. At present, studies indicate that 99% of all women who have had a cesarean will have any following children by cesarean.[1]

The possibility of uterine rupture during vaginal birth in women who have previously delivered by cesarean is extremely remote; however, the consequences of complete uterine rupture are so severe (probable hysterectomy, possible loss of mother and child) that each expectant couple and obstetrician must decide for themselves if the risk is warranted and accept responsibility for that decision. This discussion needs to take place early in pregnancy to allow time for changes in physician or hospital if necessary.

The next most common indication for cesarean birth is cephalopelvic disproportion: the head is simply too large to negotiate the mother's bony pelvis. This indication should be confirmed by pelvimetry.

Uterine dystocia or dysfunctions are another common indication. This means that the contractions are failing to bring about progress in cervical dilatation or station of the presenting part (see Chap. 7).

Fetal distress is the fourth most common reason given for performing a surgical birth. There is currently some controversy about differentiation between normal fetal stress reactions and true distress. It is undeniably true that the cesarean rate has risen sharply since electronic fetal monitoring has come into common usage. However, it is only fair to note that the climate of emphasis on a perfect outcome stimulates both constant monitoring and speed of intervention if the fetus seems stressed, for fear of malpractice suits.

Certainly the electronic fetal monitor has saved lives and improved the quality of survival for some distressed infants. The decision of when to intervene must be based on the information available at the time and the unknown quality of the stress tolerance of a given infant. Some hardy infants survive stress phases physically and developmentally unscathed, while vulnerable infants may exhibit problems at birth or later develop difficulties that may or may not be related to birth trauma. The diagnosis of fetal distress should be confirmed by fetal scalp blood sampling.

Malpresentation of the fetus includes all positions that make passage of the fetus through the pelvis difficult. This includes the breech positions as well as brow, face, shoulder, and transverse lies. If the presenting part is not engaged at the onset of labor, obstruction such as pelvic contracture or placenta previa should be suspected.

Placental problems are another indication for a cesarean delivery. This category includes abruptio placenta and placenta previa, either instance making immediate cesarean section mandatory if labor has

Table 8-2. **Indications for Cesarean Birth**

Previous cesarean birth
Cephalopelvic disproportion
Uterine dysfunctions
Fetal distress
Malpresentation
Placental problems
Maternal disease
Prolonged rupture of membranes

begun. Other placental problems include cord compression, or umbilical cords that become entangled around the baby's head so that the presenting part cannot descend.

Some maternal diseases warrant cesarean intervention. For the woman whose body is already compromised by certain diseases, the cesarean choice may be appropriate rather than the prolonged stress of labor. These diseases include diabetes (other that Class A), cardiac or hypertensive disease, severe Rh disease, pre-eclampsia, and eclampsia.

The presence of active herpesvirus in the genital tract of the mother is valid reason for cesarean birth because of the risk of infecting the newborn with a disease that is untreatable and may prove fatal. If membranes rupture in an expectant mother with active herpes genitalis, immediate cesarean birth should be planned.

Finally, prolonged rupture of membranes not culminating in the birth of the baby within 24 hours greatly increases the risk of infection in the baby. Expectant mothers should be cautioned to contact their physician and plan to be admitted to the hospital within 12 hours of rupturing membranes even if labor does not ensue.

Tests for Fetal Maturity and Well-Being

There are numerous tests available to monitor the well-being and maturity of the infant (see Chap. 7); these include pelvic ultrasound. If the initial ultrasound is done early in the pregnancy, with followup sonography late in pregnancy, an accurate date of confinement can be arrived at based on norms for head measurement and growth rate. Pelvimetry can also be measured be means of ultrasound to minimize exposure to x rays.

Amniocentesis can be performed in late pregnancy to evaluate the L–S ratio to determine fetal lung maturity.

Estriol levels in blood or urine are measured to monitor the efficiency of uteroplacental functioning. Non-stress testing is another test used to judge if the infant is still doing well (*e.g.,* when the expectant mother has gone significantly past her expected date of confinement). The woman is attached to the external electronic fetal monitor and tracings are obtained to evaluate the infant's reaction to the normal uterine activity that occurs during pregnancy. This test is used in conjunction with estriol testing and must be repeated weekly.

Getting Ready for Surgical Birth

Because of the passive roles engendered by surgical birth, too often expectant cesarean parents feel that there is nothing they can do to affect the outcome and recovery. There are some things that can be done now that involve commitment, physical conditioning, and careful nutrition. Their involvement will help the couple cope with the crisis period.

Physical Conditioning

A reminder is in order here: the body that is in good physical condition will perform better, react to stress better, and heal faster than the body in poor physical condition. This is even more crucial with a surgical birth because the stress is greater.

Prenatally, the exercises in Appendix A may be recommended. Each body part needs to be exercised and stretched to improve tone, ventilation, and flexibility. Posture and body mechanics need to be discussed, as well as the importance of proper footwear. The following suggestions are meant for the new cesarean mother to use postpartum to improve her comfort and circulation.

1. **Huffing.** *Purpose:* To help bring up phlegm from the lungs, clear the respiratory passages, and improve ventilation. *Position:* Sitting or lying. *Directions:* Take several deep breaths, followed by a loud "HA" sound. (This is like a cough, without involving the abdominal muscles or closing the throat.) Spit out any matter brought up into a tissue and discard. Repeat several times each hour for the first few postpartum days.

2. **Splinting the abdomen.** This is really a comfort measure rather than an exercise. *Purpose:* To enhance ease of movement. *Position:* When changing position, turning from side to side, or rising. *Directions:* Provide support for the incisional site by splinting with the hands (Fig 8-1) or by placing a small pillow over the abdominal area and holding in place while turning or rising. This measure may also be used for support while performing the huffing exercise above.

3. **Abdominal tightening.** *Purpose:* To improve circulation and muscle flexibility; to aid in absorption and movement of gas in the gastrointestinal tract. *Position:* Sitting or lying down. *Directions:* Place the hands over the incisional site and very gently puff the belly up, then contract the muscles by pulling in as you exhale. Repeat several times each hour for the first few days. This exercise may later be combined with pelvic tilting.

4. **Foot and ankle exercises.** *Purpose:* To improve circulation and muscle tone.
   a. *Position:* Sitting propped up in bed. *Directions:* Place both feet against a pillow placed at the foot of the bed. Alternately flex and point the feet as if walking.
   b. *Position:* Same as above. *Directions:* Inhale; while exhaling, gently slide the right leg up to a bent leg position. While inhaling again, slowly straighten it out. Repeat with other leg. Begin with only one or two leg slides, build up over several days to 5 each time. Each right leg slide counts as 1.

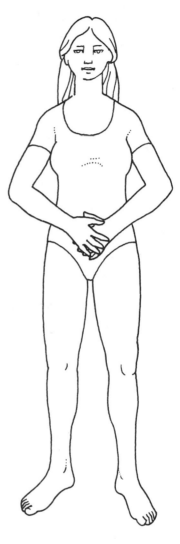

FIG. 8-1. "Splinting" the abdomen. The woman who has had a cesarean delivery may assist herself in moving or getting up (or coughing) by splinting the incision with her fingers, her wrists just anterior to the iliac crests. With permission from medical advisors, she may be encouraged to work the abdominal muscles several times daily, *very gently* contracting and releasing them while splinting with the fingers.

c. *Position:* Propped up in bed or lying down. Slide the right leg up to bent leg position. Inhale, then slide the left leg up while exhaling. Using the hands, assist the left leg to place the ankle on the right knee. *Directions:* Rotate the ankle around clockwise 10 times, then counterclockwise 10 times. Rest, take several breaths, then using the hands, help the leg to return to the both-knees-bent position. Repeat, using the other leg.

5. **Pelvic and perineal exercises.** *Purpose:* To improve circulation, muscle tone, and flexibility. *Position:* Lying in bed. *Directions:* Inhale; exhale while tightening the perineum and squeezing the

buttocks together. Use the lower back muscles to gently tilt the pelvis into a tilt position. Hold for a few seconds, inhale, and relax. Repeat three times at first, gradually building up to 5 to 10 times.

Deep breathing, shoulder rotations, and head rotations as well as frequent moving around in bed should all be encouraged.

Nutrition

Another important consideration when preparing for the stress of cesarean birth is maintenance of excellent nutrition. This topic may have been covered in classes that the couple attended for a previous birth, or by their own health care provider. Nevertheless it warrants discussion to improve motivation in late pregnancy. Helping couples to assess their own eating patterns is most useful because they will base their diet plans on their own preferences. One way to do this is to have them fill out dietary intake sheets for 3 full days, with foods eaten divided into columns for the basic food groups. These can be assessed at a later class, and each couple can see for themselves if they are meeting their own food needs. If the effects of good nutrition are related to levels of wellness or recovery speed, motivation and interest will be increased.

Because of bowel manipulation that will take place at the time of surgery, it is an excellent preparation if the mother will eat a diet high in fiber beginning about 4 weeks before her due date. She can do this by including high-fiber foods such as celery, whole grains, or fresh pineapple in her diet, as well as bran. The bran may be taken as cereal (be sure it is 100 % bran, however, such as Wheatena or Crackling Bran), as bran flakes, or as tablets available at a health food store. The woman needs to be encouraged to keep taking her prenatal vitamins, and some physicians include extra vitamin E (100 mg/day) as well.

In the postpartum period, the woman should return to her bran intake as soon as she returns to a regular diet while still in the hospital. Empirical data suggests a much earlier return to normal bowel function when this regimen is followed.

During the extended postpartum period, the new mother needs to continue to eat a well-balanced high-protein diet, and to continue her vitamins with the possible addition of iron and vitamin C to promote healing.

Hospital Admission

Couples should be encouraged to tour the hospital unit where the birth will take place. At the same time they can preregister in the admitting office, fill out admission forms, and ask questions about hospital policy such as visiting hours, rooming in, sibling visitation, father presence in the cesarean birth room and so forth. A request can be made at this time to have another cesarean mother assigned as a roommate if possible.

If arrangements have been made for the admission to take place on the morning of surgery, the expectant mother will need to come in to have blood drawn and to have a chest x-ray a day or two prior to the scheduled admission; otherwise this will be done on the day of admission. The obstetrical resident will take a detailed history and perform the admission physical examination. Permission forms for the surgery and anesthesia will have to be signed and witnessed.

The evening before the birth the anesthesiologist will interview the expectant mother. This is the time to discuss choices in anesthesia. (Even though this was discussed earlier in the pregnancy with the obstetrician, it needs to be clarified with the anesthesiologist.) Epidural anesthesia is usually the preferred choice if it is available. Because administration of epidural anesthesia requires considerable expertise on the part of the anesthesiologist, it is unwise to insist on this choice unless the anesthesiologist is entirely comfortable with its use. Spinal anesthesia also allows for the mother to be awake and to see her child as soon as it is delivered.

General anesthesia may be the appropriate choice if speed is necessary (unlikely in the planned cesarean birth), if the mother prefers to be asleep, or if some physical abnormality in the mother precludes the use of conduction anesthesia.

The anesthesiologist will want to know of any past experiences with analgesics or anesthetics, including untoward or allergic reactions. Occasionally, expectant couples are hesitant to ask questions or state preferences to the anesthesiologist because he is usually a stranger to them. It may help if they remember that the anesthesiologist is a skilled physician whose expertise they are hiring. As educated consumers, they have a duty to inquire and to discuss their preferences.

Either the night before or on the morning of the birth, the expectant mother will be asked to shower with a bacteriostatic cleanser and will have her abdominal and suprapubic hair shaved. Before being taken to the anesthesia room, a Foley catheter will be inserted to keep the bladder empty during the birth, and an intravenous infusion will be started. The woman can request that a vein on the forearm or the back of the hand be used so that she will still be able to move her elbow and hand. She may be given an antacid to neutralize stomach acids in case of regurgitation or vomiting. Her rings will be removed or taped in place. If she needs her glasses to see her baby clearly, she should be reminded to take them along. She will receive some premedication that will make her somewhat sleepy, and dry up secretions in the nose and mouth. Sometime later she will be moved by stretcher to the anesthesia room.

If epidural or spinal anesthesia is used, the mother will be asked to curl up on her side around her baby ("C" or "rainbow" position) to increase intervertebral space and allow easier visualization and administration of the anesthetic. If the father is to be present, he should ask to accompany her. He can remind her to relax and perhaps use rhythmic chest breathing while uncomfortable procedures are being done. He can hold her hand and offer reassurance throughout.

After the regional anesthesia has been administered, the woman will lose sensation in her legs and up to just below the rib cage. Her legs may feel numb or warm. She will feel the movement when she is moved onto the table.

She should be prepared to see a number of persons in the surgery room who may be strangers to her. Other than her obstetrician and the anesthesiologist, the members of the childbirth team may include the hospital resident or residents, the scrub nurse and one or two circulating nurses, the nursery nurse, and the pediatrician or pediatric resident.

The fetal heart tones are monitored, and a pillow may be placed under one hip to displace the weight of the gravid uterus from the inferior vena cava. A grounding plate will be attached to the woman's leg for use with the electric cautery that will close off small blood vessels during the surgical birth.

The abdomen is washed with a bacteriostatic cleanser, then the sterile drapes are placed around the incisional area and attached to form a screen near the mother's head. This keeps her from looking directly into the incision and limits the number of bacteria from her nasopharyngeal tract that reach the operative site. The father, if he is present, will sit next to her shoulders and can speak softly to her. He is likewise screened from watching the operation.

The skin incision will usually be a low transverse ("smile" or "bikini") incision unless there is need for great speed. If the mother has a previous classical scar, the obstetrician may choose to enter the skin through the old site, excising the old scar; this does not affect the placement of the uterine incision. Next, the incision is made through fatty tissue, with small blood vessels being cauterized. The parents may expect to hear the buzzing sound made by the cautery. The muscle layer is then separated and the uterus exposed. The bladder flap is peeled back and retracted, and a low transverse incision is made into the uterus.

The parents will hear the sound of suctioning as amniotic fluid is suctioned and the uterine muscle retracted. The baby is then delivered up through the incision. The parents may watch in a mirror if available, or the father may be invited to stand up to witness the birth. He can then describe the event to the mother and identify the sex for her.

The mother should expect to feel pressure or tugging sensations, but no pain. If she feels dizziness or nausea, this should be reported to the anesthesiologist and oxygen may be administered.

The baby is assessed, and the nose and mouth suctioned. The cord is clamped and cut. He or she is then placed in a heated bassinet and dried thoroughly. As cesarean infants are likely to have more fluid in their noses and mouths than vaginally born infants, suctioning will probably be continued, with administration of oxygen.

The father, if he is present, may be invited to watch as the baby receives its initial physical exam from the pediatrician. He may then have his child placed in his arms to present to his wife. If he is not present, the circulating or nursery nurse can take over this function. A request should be made to delay the instillation of eye drops until a later time.

Meanwhile, the placenta is manually removed, the uterus again suctioned, and the repair begun. Following this the wound is repaired, including muscle and fatty layers, and finally the skin. The skin incision may be closed with clips, much like staples, or with sutures. The incision is dressed, and the new mother is cleaned up and taken to the recovery room until her vital signs are stable. The baby is usually taken to the nursery for a bath and temperature check. If all is well and hospital policy permits, the baby will then rejoin the parents in the recovery room for some quiet time together.

Postpartum Care

In the recovery room the mother's pulse and blood pressure, as well as a fundal height and lochia, will continue to be monitored. The new mother may feel somewhat groggy from preoperative medication. Gradually, as the anesthesia begins to wear off, the mother will begin to regain feeling in her toes. She should be encouraged to wriggle her toes and feet around to improve circulation and speed recovery. As sensation returns she should request pain medication if she needs it; this will make moving around and handling her baby easier. If the baby is to be nursed, this may be begun in the recovery room as well, with the father there to help with positioning.

Once the anesthesia has worn off and the vital signs are stable, the new mother returns to her room. The IV and the Foley catheter will probably remain in place for at least 24 hours.

Probably the major cause of postpartum pain is gas formation, which must be absorbed by the gut and expelled. The absorption and movement of gas within the gastrointestinal tract can be assisted by gentle contraction and relaxation of the abdominal musculature, pelvic rocking, leg sliding, and early ambulation. In order to minimize additional gas formation there are a few precautions the new mother should observe once she is placed on a liquid diet. She should avoid using straws (because more air is likely to be swallowed) and iced liquids for a few days. Warm liquids such as broth or tea are preferable. For many woman, milk may cause gas and cramping. Later, gas-forming vegetables such as those in the bean, pea, or cabbage families should be avoided.

The new mother may need a reminder to "huff" and deep breathe every hour or so to assist in bringing up phlegm and to improve ventilation. She should also "walk" her feet against a pillow placed at the foot of her bed (see Getting Ready for Surgical Birth, Foot and Ankle Exercises). These and other exercises are all for improvement of circulation and in preparation for getting out of bed. The woman can be reminded how to splint the abdomen with her hands or a pillow for turning or rising and to keep a side rail up to assist her. The first time out of bed should not be attempted without the assistance of a nurse. The mother turns to her side, moves her feet over the side of the bed and sits up with the help of the nurse, with legs dangling over the side. She pauses, deep breathes, splints the abdomen, then, with the help of the nurse, stands up straight. That first walk to the bathroom may seem long, but the nurse will assist, then help the new mother back into her bed.

If the baby is in the intensive care nursery, the mother may request to be taken in a wheelchair to see and to touch. Presumably the father will have done this already and will give the infant as much touching and holding as possible.

If the mother is nursing, she may need help with positioning at first. The "football" position is a good one, with the baby's body lying with its feet under the mother's arm and the head next to the breast. Or the mother may lie on her side with the infant on a pillow next to her in reach of her nipple. Another position might be to place a pillow over the incisional area and rest the baby on the pillow.

A reminder is made to cut down on pain medication if nursing. A good time to receive pain medication if needed is right after a feeding session so that the amount left in the mother's system is low by the time of the next feeding. The obstetrician or pediatrician should be consulted. In many cases an oral, less potent drug may be ordered once bowel functioning returns.

In hospitals where rooming in is available, this can usually be started as soon as the mother has gained some ease in moving around and handling the infant.

The return to a regular diet is usually cause for celebration and a psychological boost as well. The bran taken prenatally should be started again at this time because it gives a high-bulk, soft stool that is easily passed.

The cesarean mother is usually ready to be discharged from the hospital after 5 to 7 days. She will need help at home for a time, while she concentrates on her own recovery and on her new baby. If she was discharged early, she will need an appointment with her physician at 1 week postpartum to remove skin clips or sutures.

Father-Attended Cesarean Birth

Parents today do not want to be excluded from an emotionally rewarding, joyful event in their lives. Although father (coach) attendance in the cesarean birth room is not yet an option in many places, there are some strategies that couples can employ to make the possibility more likely.

The couple should start early in the pregnancy to make their desire to be together known. They can explore with their obstetrician how he feels about father participation. If their obstetrician does not wish to have the father present, the couple will need to decide if their desire is strong enough to warrant a change of obstetrician, if there is a choice. The same holds true for the hospital. If the chosen hospital does not allow father participation, all avenues should be explored to encourage them to change their policy, or a change of hospital may be considered. Help should be sought from their own obstetrician. Hospital administration should be contacted. The couple should make their requests politely but firmly. They should try to enlist the administration's aid with their mutual problem. They can seek out and discuss their desires with the anesthesiologists. If state laws are quoted to support exclusion, they can find out if such laws exist (probably not). If lack of space is the problem, they can find out what other hospitals have done to overcome this obstacle. Finally, if permission is granted, they should get it from administration and *they should get it in writing* and take it with them at the time of admission.

If the father is to be allowed into the cesarean birth room, it is essential that he understand exactly what is expected, where he may sit, and when and under what circumstances movement around the room is possible. He needs the same information as the expectant mother who will be awake for the delivery about the procedures and the sounds he will hear, such as the suctioning of the uterine cavity.

Usually the father will change and gown in the changing room before entering. He needs to know that the hospital will not be responsible for his valuables, and arrange to leave them at home or with a friend or family member. When allowed, he may stay with the expectant mother while the spinal or epidural anesthetic is being administered. He may usually hold her hand, and offer a calm, supportive voice to remind her to use her relaxation and controlled breathing while the needle is being inserted. When she is moved into the surgery room, he must be escorted to his place by a member of the nursing staff, and remain seated there until or unless he is escorted elsewhere. Usually this will be next to his wife's shoulders where he can talk softly to her and touch her reassuringly on the shoulder or arm. He will be screened from watching the surgery itself, just as she is. Often at the time of the birth, the obstetrician will invite him to stand up to see his child emerge, wet and slippery, to draw its first breath. He can then be the one to describe the event to the new mother and identify the sex for her. He must understand, however, that he still must stay where he is and not move around the room. After the infant is suctioned and the pediatrician has begun the initial physical examination, he may invite the new father to come watch. In this case, the circulating nurse escorts the father over to the bassinet. After the pediatrician has completed his task and the infant is scored either on the Apgar or Brazelton scale, the new father may be given the baby to hold and to present to his wife. He needs to hold it near to her face so she can see it, and unwrap the body and limbs for her observation without allowing the baby to chill. If her arms are strapped for IV, blood pressure apparatus, and so forth, she will be unable to reach for her child. In this case, the baby can be held against her cheek so she can nuzzle, stroke and smell the unique smell of the new born. As in the regular birth room, request should be made that eye drop instillation be delayed until the parents have had the opportunity to establish this first bonding contact.

The coach will need to remember as clearly as possible the events of the birth, because the new mother will probably have only fragmentary recollection owing to premedication. The couple will need to talk the event through later to help the woman fit her coach's recollection of the birth into her memory of the birth. This helps to keep the continuity in the adjustment from being pregnant to being a new parent. If permission is granted, photographs taken of parents and baby in the delivery room can clarify the event. If not, they may be allowed in the recovery room if the baby is present.

For fathers who must be excluded from the birth room, the planning and working-through process can be encouraged by attending cesarean birth classes, by touring the hospital unit, by seeking information, along with his mate, about cesarean births, and by remaining as physically close as is permitted during the admission, presurgical, and postsurgical periods. By taking as active a part as he possibly can, his spouse is assured of his continuing interest and concern, even when they must be physically separate.

Gradually, hospitals and obstetricians will become less fearful. There is no evidence of an increased number of malpractice suits as a result of father attendance in the cesarean birth room, any more than when fathers were first allowed to attend their wives in labor rooms and delivery rooms a few years ago. On the contrary, many, if not most, lawsuits seem to result from the feeling that the doctor and hospital did not do their best in a given situation, or that the parents were not given due respect or consideration. Fathers who attend cesarean births seem invariably impressed with the professional competence and technical expertise of the obstetrician, anesthesiologist, and operating room staff. They feel included and emotionally supported. It seems logical that this situation would be likely to decrease rather than to increase the number of malpractice suits.

Vaginal Delivery After Cesarean

Although the majority of practitioners presently prefer to repeat the cesarean birth, a growing number are willing to consider vaginal delivery under proper conditions.

Careful selection of candidates for vaginal delivery is mandatory. The previous cesarean should have been done for a nonrepeating reason such as fetal distress, and the expectant mother must have no current or additional reason for cesarean. Women with a classical incision scar on the uterus run a greater risk of complete uterine rupture and should not attempt vaginal delivery.

The expectant parents need to be counseled about possible risks involved and to understand that there is a possibility that another cesarean will be necessary if difficulties evolve.

There must be a single fetus with the vertex presenting, weighing less than 8.8 pounds.

The expectant mother must agree to enter the hospital when labor begins so that she may be carefully monitored throughout labor. Reserve blood supplies, and emergency equipment and personnel for surgery should be immediately available, and the obstetrician physically present throughout labor. The anesthesiologist and pediatrician should be alerted and available in case of emergency.

If these criteria are met, the American College of Obstetricians and Gynecologists Committee on Obstetrics has determined that ". . . many women who have had a cesarean birth may safely be considered for vaginal delivery."[1]

References

1. American College of Obstetricians and Gynecologists: Vaginal delivery after cesarean. News Release (Washington, DC), Feb 24, 1982
2. Allinson E: Lecture presented at Maternity Center Association, New York, 1981
3. Highley B, Mercer R: Safeguarding the laboring woman's sense of control. American Journal of Maternal Child Nursing 3(1):39–41, 1978
4. Young D, Mahan C: Unnecessary Cesareans: Ways to Avoid Them. Minneapolis, International Childbirth Education Association, 1980

9

Preparation for the Postpartum and New Parenting Experience

Immediate Postpartum

Physical Recovery

Involution of the Generative Organs

If the newly delivered mother looks down at her abdomen, she can observe the globular-shaped fundus about halfway between her symphysis and her umbilicus. **Palpation** by herself or the nurse in massaging the fundus shows the whole abdominal area as well as the uterus to be extremely sensitive after the exertions of labor.

The uterus remains at approximately the same height for about 48 hours, then begins to shrink down so quickly that by the tenth **postpartum** day the fundus can no longer be felt; it has regained its position as a pelvic organ. This shrinking takes place by a series of uterine contractions, noticeable to the new mother, which are commonly referred to as "afterpains." She may be prepared for this by a discussion of the processes by which the female body recovers from the stresses of childbearing. Because of the relationship of nursing and the occurrence of afterpains, it should be explained that the same hormone that allows the milk to "let down" causes this shrinking of the uterus. This reassures her that her body is continuing to function normally in the involuntary process. She also needs to know that these cramps will not continue forever, but will subside as the uterus returns to normal size. The multipara experiences more marked cramping than the primiparous woman, because her uterus is inclined to be more lax and requires more vigorous contraction.

The **lochia** is red and plentiful for the first 2 to 2½ weeks and seems to the mother rather like a heavy menstrual period. It gradually becomes brownish, more serous, and eventually whitish. The new mother should be reminded that her body has taken on a greater volume of blood during her pregnancy so that she will not fear the blood loss. The lochia rubra can be described as "like menstural bleeding," that is, without large clots, although there are bits of tissue present. The endometrium heals by sloughing off the superficial layer of cells and necrotic tissue from the placental site, with concurrent regrowth of healthy new epithelium underneath.[7] The mother should expect to have some lochia for about 4½ weeks.

The perineum feels sore, even if an episiotomy has not been done, because of the tremendous stretching it has undergone. For the first few days the mother experiences some discomfort when she sits and may be frightened, if she has stitches, to urinate or defecate. Much of this discomfort can be alleviated or avoided if she can be persuaded to begin her perineal contraction exercises (Appendix A) within the first hour and to continue to do them every hour for the first few days. The resultant increase in circulation helps to prevent edema and stiffness.

Because the women in prenatal classes tend to wince when episiotomy is mentioned, the childbirth educator might explain why an immediate return to this exercise is important by using a nonthreatening example from another body area. The example often chosen is the wrist. The instructor might suggest that the class imagine that a cut on the wrist is carefully protected from movement for a few days. Then it becomes difficult to move the wrist at all because of muscle stiffness. On the other hand, if movement is continued, slowly at first, there is a gradual return to comfort without added limitation of motion.

Other measures to increase comfort include tailor sitting (see Fig. 5-5,*A*), which places the weight on the ischial tuberosities rather than on the perineum. This position is more comfortable than trying to avoid pressure on stitches by sitting on one buttock, which causes the perineal area to twist, or on a rubber ring, unless the ring is carefully placed. The tailor position is also ideal for holding and feeding an infant. A pillow on the lap supports the mother's arm while she is holding the baby. Finally, the perineal pad should not be held too tightly against the perineum. One method to ensure proper placement and avoid friction against the stitches is to attach the pad to the underpants with a pin in the front only. The pants hold the pad in place without pulling upward. When the mother is at home, the new pads with a sticky side that attaches to the underpants are ideal.

Specific care and comfort measures for perineal care, such as ice packs, heat lamps, or **sitz baths**, may differ according to the hospital or physician and will be explained to the new mother by the hospital nurse.

Abdominal Wall

After childbirth the abdominal wall is lax and flabby, and may remain so unless the mother does some type of physical fitness exercise to regain muscle tone. In our automated society, although the new mother works hard and is physically tired, her abdominal muscles are not ordinarily called upon to perform more than minimally in the course of her day. Occasionally a **diastasis recti** results. During the first days, some abdominal breathing exercises are sufficient to begin the process of regaining muscle tone. Unless contraindicated by her physician or midwife, these can be followed over a period of time by abdominal isometrics, head raising, pelvic rocking, leg raising, and eventually sit-ups (see Appendix A). The new mother should be cautioned to begin slowly and gradually increase the amount of exercise each day as her physical recovery continues.

Although the sleep-deprived new mother may not get around to the reinstitution of a regularly scheduled exercise session, the perineal and abdominal tightening can be hooked into some frequently performed activity to ensure that these two critical exercises get done. For example, if the mother can accustom herself to tightening the perineum and the abdominal muscles every time she turns on the water faucet, muscle tone will be regained quickly. The abdominal wall should be back to normal in about 6 to 7 weeks.

Urinary Tract

During the birth process, the bladder and urethra undergo a certain amount of unavoidable trauma. This results in some loss of sensitivity to fluid pressure from within and may cause bladder retention because the new mother is unaware of the urge to urinate for the first postpartum day or so. She needs to be reminded to listen to the cues her body is giving her, especially since this early postpartum period is marked by a **diuresis** as the body rids itself of the excess fluid retained in the course of the pregnancy.

Gastrointestinal Tract

Constipation is extremely common in the immediate postpartum period for several reasons. The anus has become slightly less sensitive because of the tremendous pressure it has undergone. In addition, there is a slight slowing down of intestinal **peristalsis**, and the mother's lax abdominal muscles are not of much assistance in promoting defecation. The mother may be afraid to exert any pressure because of the still sore episiotomy or hemorrhoids. Also, although she is thirsty and drinks a lot, the diuretic action means that fluid is quickly voided, and the intestinal contents may become dried out and hard.

A mild **cathartic** or an enema is frequently ordered on the third day if the mother has not returned to normal bowel functioning. In the later postpartum period, the mother may request a stool softener from her physician and should be encouraged to eat a well-balanced diet that includes enough roughage. Mild exercising also helps to relieve constipation.

The Breasts

During pregnancy the breasts have been prepared for lactation by the combined influences of estrogen, progesterone, and **chorion somato-**

mammotropin, which also inhibit untimely production of milk. At delivery, these hormone levels drop abruptly. When the infant is put to the breast and stimulates the nipple, the pituitary gland releases another hormone, **prolactin**, which initiates milk production.

The suckling of the infant during nursing stimulates the release of oxytocin from the **neurohypophysis**. This hormone causes the contraction of the myoepithelial cells that line the alveoli, propelling the fluid forward into the lactiferous ducts behind the areola. This is the well-known "let down" reflex and feels to the mother like a tingling and filling up of her breasts. Because oxytocin also stimulates contraction of the uterus, the new mother feels sharp cramping at the start of each nursing period for the first few days. She should be reassured that this is nature's way of returning her body to its prepregnant state.

Until the true milk comes in, the fluid that the infant gets from the breasts is colostrum. This valuable first food provides protein, minerals, vitamins A and E, and nitrogen in an easily digestible form. Its cathartic properties help the infant eliminate the **meconium** that fills its gastro-intestinal tract at birth.

On about the third postpartum day, perhaps sooner if the infant was put to breast immediately postdelivery, the breasts become tender and **engorged**. The mother experiences some pain and throbbing and notes that her breasts have become enlarged and hot with distended veins. A few women run a slight temperature during this period. In the primipara the "coming in" of the milk is likely to be quite stormy, and the breast skin may become so distended that it has a sheen to it. If she is unprepared for this, she may imagine that nursing will always be like this and wonder if it is worth it. She needs to be reassured that the discomfort will disappear by about the seventh to tenth day. Frequent nursing can help to alleviate the discomfort. A supportive brassiere, which can be worn even during the night while the engorgement persists, is also helpful.

Another problem that the new nursing mother often encounters during the engorgement period is leakage of milk. If nursing pads are insufficient, some mothers cut a sanitary pad into thirds and insert it into the brassiere. The sticky-tape side adheres to the brassiere to hold it in place. Again, the mother needs reassurance that the engorgement period is limited or she is likely to imagine that nursing will always be messy.

To further complicate matters, the breast may become so distended that the infant cannot grasp the nipple and chews on the areola instead (which hurts). **Expressing** some of the milk immediately prior to nursing can allow the infant to find the nipple more easily. Another alternative is to begin the nursing session with a nipple shield, removing the shield after the areola has softened somewhat.

As long as the mother nurses, prolactin is released from the anterior pituitary to stimulate further milk production, and oxytocin causes it to be let down. If the milk supply seems inadequate at times, more frequent nursing with its attendant increased stimulation of the prolactin release will build it up again. Interference with the let down is a more common problem, because the let down is easily influenced by psychological elements such as anxiety or tension.

In prenatal discussions of breast-feeding, it is wise to keep suggestions few and simple. Overloading the expectant mother with specific suggestions makes it difficult to get the main points across. Consider offering a few very general suggestions, being sure she understands the relationship between supply and nursing demand as well as the importance of psychological support, adequate rest, nourishment, and fluid. The labor coach can be enlisted to help here. If the woman is planning to breast-feed, she should be encouraged to purchase a book about nursing for general advice and for middle-of-the-night consultation. One highly recommended book for this purpose is *The Complete Book of Breastfeeding*, which is available in paperback.[4]

If the mother is not planning to nurse her infant, she is given an injection containing estrogen or testosterone immediately after delivery to inhibit the milk production. If the breasts become engorged in spite of this, the mother should know that in the absence of nursing or expression of the milk, they will soon dry up. Comfort measures include a supportive brassiere, temperature (milk supply is inhibited when circulation is restricted, so cold is preferable to heat), restriction of fluids, and aspirin.

Weight Loss

With the expulsion of the uterine contents, there is a weight loss of about 12 to 13 pounds. During the first week there is a further loss of about 5 pounds as diuresis and **diaphoresis** dispose of the extra fluid that had been retained during the pregnancy.

The nursing mother can expect, if her diet is sensible, to lose the remaining 10 pounds or so over a period of the next few months. The nonnursing mother, who is not expending the extra calories required for milk production, may have to regulate her caloric intake if she desires to lose more weight.

Emotional Changes

Immediately after the birth, the new mother feels physically exhausted but experiences an emotional "high." The need to share her joy often interferes with her need for rest. Too often she phones everyone she knows to invite them to visit her in the hospital and view the newborn, only to spend the time of the visit wishing they would go. To protect the new mother from too much exertion at first, some hospitals have stringent visiting policies.

Besides a feeling of satisfaction if the mother feels she handled the labor and birth well, or of disappointment if she feels she did not, the new mother is concerned with her new body image. If she accepted the changes of pregnancy in a wholesome manner, chances are good that the discomforts of the postpartum period will not distress her unduly. The woman who was unable to accept her pregnant body—who constantly fretted about her "ugly" appearance and who considered herself "gross"—may have a rude awakening if she is unprepared for her body appearance in the immediate postnatal period. Her breasts may be sore and leaking unexpectedly, her belly flabby and sagging, her perineum sore or itching as the stitches resolve themselves, and the lochia ever-present. If she has been counting on wearing her prepregnancy clothing home from the hospital, she may be sadly disappointed.

The parents need to know that things have usually settled down by about 3 weeks; the lochia has lessened or disappeared, the milk let down has become more predictable, and the soreness from the episiotomy has gone. The woman who loved being pregnant, who felt completely realized, and who reveled in the signs of her gravid state may feel a sense of loss when her child is born. This need to grieve for the loss of the pregnant state may hinder her in her task of transition from "nest to nurturer" in the first month.[3] Sometimes this transition is made more difficult if the father or visitors transfer all of their attention to the new baby and ignore the person who is now a new mother. In the psychically healthy woman, this feeling of loss gives way as she interacts and becomes absorbed with her infant.

If a realistic picture has been presented to her in prenatal classes, it is easier for the new mother to accept herself as she is rather than as she expected to be postnatally. The childbirth educator must stress that these discomforts are proof that the body is getting on with its tasks of involution and nurturing.

Extended Postpartum

Physical and Physiological States

The reparation processes that were begun in the immediate postpartum continue during the fourth trimester. The uterus, which had shrunk down into the pelvis again by about the tenth postpartal day, continues to shrink until it attains its usual nonpregnant size at about 5 to 6 weeks.[7] At the same time, regeneration of the **endometrium** is taking place. By the end of the third week the entire endometrium is restored, except for the placental site, which takes up to 6 weeks.[7]

The vagina, which has undergone tremendous stretching during the birth process, presents a smooth, cavernous appearance in the early puerperium. Gradually it shrinks down in size, although it rarely returns to its prepregnant condition. The **rugae** begin to reappear about the third postpartum week.

The menstrual period will probably return in 1 to 2 months if the mother is not nursing her infant. With the nursing mother it may take longer to return, depending somewhat upon how fully the infant is being nursed. The mother should be warned, however, that ovulation precedes menstruation most of the time. The fact that she has not yet menstruated is not a reliable test for fertility.

Many women notice hair loss in the months following delivery. This is a result of the slowing down of the rapid growth period during pregnancy.

Emotional State

The Mother's Needs

The dependency needs and emotional lability that were characteristic of the third trimester extend into the fourth trimester as well when the new mother is redefining herself in her new role. If the early weeks are unlike the fantasy she had created or if she does not feel as she believes mothers should feel, she may be sad. Her need to prove herself a good mother may cause her to become so preoccupied with the infant that all else is excluded, even her mate. If her image of a good mother includes a sparkling house, freshly ironed laundry, and gourmet meals, she may further exhaust herself attempting to live up to her ideal, then wonder why she is unhappy. Concurrently, her body is adjusting to new hormonal levels, because the pregnancy levels to which she had become accustomed have been abruptly withdrawn.

The new mother's needs for nurturing and for dependable companionship are vitally important, yet her strong need to prove her capability may hinder her from seeking or accepting this kind of support.

How the mother feels she managed her labor also influences how she feels about her nurturing abilities. If she did not live up to her expectation or if intervention was necessary, she has less confidence in her own competence as a mother.

In prenatal class the childbirth educator can give some anticipatory guidance. Giving a realistic picture of the puerperium reduces feelings of anxiety when things are not going smoothly. There are several ways to create a supportive milieu for the new mother. One way is by enlisting the aid of the expectant father and explaining the problem to him. A lateral support system might be established by actively helping prenatal classmates keep in touch with each other. This can be done by giving out a class roster with phone numbers or planning a new parent get-together with the new babies 1 month after the last due date. Finally, the childbirth educator herself can phone new parents to see how things are going and make herself available for phone consultation.

Help at Home

The expectant parents should think about the need for help and rest by discussing the kinds of help that might be available. If the baby's father can take vacation time or paternity leave, then the couple can become acquainted with the newborn and adjust to their new roles together. Household tasks can be shared or neglected.

Often a grandmother is available and can give wonderful support, but the couple should consider what their relationship is with this person. If the new parents are going to feel threatened in developing their own parenting skills, perhaps the grandmother should delay the visit a few weeks.

Another alternative is hired help. The couple should decide what it is they want help with and be sure that this is understood by the helper. The usual choice is help with housework, cooking, and shopping so that the mother can rest and concentrate on the baby. Some couples choose a baby nurse, which can be fine if the nurse is skilled at nurturing and will help the new mother to learn. But if the helper, be it baby nurse or baby's grandmother, takes control of decisions about the baby, it hinders the development of the new mother's nurturing skills. She needs protection from this kind of assistance.

By accepting the fact that the mother should rest and let the housework go for a while, the childbirth educator helps her to feel right about doing this.

The teacher should be aware that the expectant parents do not fully integrate this teaching until they have their child. Couples expecting their first child are unable to imagine a time when fatigue overrides all other considerations for weeks on end. It can make this difficult period go more smoothly, however, if they have been forewarned and understand that this is a normal component of the new parenting experience, and that it is time limited.

The Father's Needs

Pregnancy evokes feelings of protectiveness in most men, as well as anxiety about the burden of being sole provider. These feelings are viewed as appropriate and acceptable in our society. If the protectiveness develops into nurturant emotions, however, these emotions may be considered feminine and inappropriate. For this reason, such feelings may be denied by the expectant father.

Expectant fathers who choose to involve themselves by coming to childbirth classes and nurturing their wives in labor may be more willing to admit to these feelings and to share them with each other. By discussing the range of normal emotions in childbirth classes, the instructor can show her acceptance of a father in a nurturing role and encourage lateral sharing and support.

If the expectant father feels that his nurturant emotions are unmanly, he may detach himself emotionally from the pregnancy. He may involve himself in a new hobby, become absorbed in physical preparations for the child, or accept a new and demanding job. Such a reaction is often defended by citing anxiety about the new role of sole provider, which is seen as acceptable. If this all-too-typical mode of adaptive behavior continues into the parenting period, the stereotyped American family develops: matricentral, father absent most of the waking time, paternally deprived children.[1]

To help the expectant father who would like to become an active, involved parent anticipate negative social pressures from male peers, extended family, and people at work, Heise has suggested that the following questions be brought up for class discussion:

- How do I see myself? What is my concept of masculine involvement with my wife and child in the family setting? What will others think of me in this role?
- Does my wife accept my role as an involved father? Will she support me in the event of social pressures? Do we have a working understanding of the difference between passive breadwinner role and father in an involved aggressive role in the family?
- What arrangements must be made relevant to my job?[6]

How much involvement the father would like in his parenting role and how much his wife would like him to have must be worked out between themselves. The degree of satisfaction depends more upon mutual agreement than upon how much responsibility the father actually accepts.

Many new fathers find it difficult to cope with their still-moody mates. The emotional lability that was present during pregnancy continues well into the puerperium, sometimes for many months. This moodiness is overlaid with fatigue in the early weeks as well as the normal stress that accompanies family readjustments. The new father may have been willing to overlook this behavior as a part of pregnancy, but unwilling to go on overlooking it once the pregnancy is over. He may feel that the new mother is being unreasonable and that it is time she "shaped up." Also, he often does not have a place to express these views, which adds to his frustration and guilt feelings.

New fathers are also frequently concerned about loss of freedom. If the baby is their first, the new parents cannot come and go as freely as before. In addition, the new mother is so involved with the infant that fathers often feel left out. In class the childbirth educator should stress the importance of making plans to leave the baby with some other responsible adult for a "baby break" within the first month. Both parents need a breather and will return refreshed. Each may have been so intent upon the infant that they have neglected their relationship with each other. The outing need not be an elaborate affair—even an afternoon walk alone will do—but they should plan to do something alone. It might be suggested that they go out to dinner to celebrate the newborn's 1-month birthday!

Sexuality

The last thing the couple in the last trimester may expect is a problem with their sex lives. They may or may not have been coping well with the mechanical inconveniences of advancing pregnancy, but at least they see this as a time-limited phenomenon. They often wonder about a return to their usual sex practices, but seldom voice this question, thinking it "too trivial" or inappropriate in childbirth classes. The childbirth class may be their only real resource, however, because their physician may seem too busy or inaccessible.

Most childbirth educators are not qualified to be sex counselors; however, it is appropriate to give information about the physical and emotional elements that may affect a happy return to coital pleasure. Also, bringing up the topic in class identifies sexuality as a legitimate area of concern.

Physically, the female body is in a state of steroid deprivation because the ovaries do not return to normal steroid production until the ovulatory cycle begins again. For the first few months the vaginal mucosa has a thin, light pink, smooth appearance, and the woman is probably not able to lubricate as she normally would when sexually aroused. This condition can be expected to persist for several months, more in the nursing mother. This dryness can be distressing for the couple, especially since some males measure female response by ability to lubricate. The woman can use either a water-soluble lubricating gel (not Vaseline—it is not water soluble and requires vigorous washing to remove) or contraceptive cream. Ideally, it should be applied in advance of lovemaking because it is cold.

Once the lochia stops and the episiotomy is healed, usually about 3 weeks, there is no physiological reason why vaginal intercourse cannot safely be resumed. Not all couples are ready at 3 weeks, however. Either partner may suffer fears about penetration. Both are concerned about causing possibly permanent damage if coitus is resumed too soon.[10]

If the couple have been actively relieving each other's sexual tensions in the pregnancy period by methods other than vaginal intercourse, they will probably continue to do so in the puerperium until they are both ready to resume vaginal **coitus.** They need to understand the mutuality of the problem and to be encouraged to resolve it together. Practically, the childbirth educator can restate couple's mutual need for reassurance that they are still sexually desirable (see Sexual Activity: Controversy and Concern, Chap. 5), and again mention modes of sexual expression other than vaginal intercourse, such as stroking or fondling (commonly known as foreplay). When they do return to intercourse, a position in which the female can control the depth of penetration, such as female superior or side by side, reduces fears about injury.

In addition to problems of fear of injury or pain, constant fatigue, and fear of awakening the infant, the nursing mother may find that her breasts spurt milk during orgasm, a fact that either partner may find unattractive. The couple may use a towel to solve this problem, or the mother can wear her brassiere during lovemaking. Interestingly, in spite of this additional embarrassment, the nursing mothers in Masters and Johnson's study reported an earlier return of erotic interest and an earlier return to coitus than did the nonnursing group.[10]

If the woman does not wish to conceive again immediately, she must consult her physician about contraception. Her prepregnant form of contraception must be reevaluated in the light of her postpartal state. If, for example, she used oral contraceptives, her physician may prefer that she have one normal ovulatory cycle before she resumes taking the pill. The nursing mother must also consider the fact that the pill can interfere with milk production. If she used a diaphragm, the size should be checked because of the changes in cervical size brought about by the pregnancy. An intrauterine device (IUD) may be the method of choice, but she must make this decision in consultation with her physician. Usually this discussion of contraception takes place at the postpartum checkup 3 to 6 weeks after delivery. If the couple wishes to return to intercourse before this time, however, the physician can be consulted by phone for an interim form of contraception.

Family Integration

The first task of parenting is identification of the newborn. The parents must be able to see for themselves that the baby is here, it is theirs, and it is well or otherwise. All other integration tasks follow. If the mother has been anesthetized, the whole beginning of parenting is delayed until she has seen the baby.

Childbirth educators are in a unique position. They have the opportunity to influence the infant's early integration into the family by helping the expectant parents decide on priorities. The myth of instant parenthood must be exploded, because many new parents fear that there is something wrong with them if they do not feel an immediate, overwhelming rush of parental feeling when they first see their newborn. Parenting behavior and parental love develop through touching and caring for the newborn (following identification), and for this reason it is worthwhile stressing the importance of early physical contact. Unless there is a valid *medical* contraindication, they should be encouraged to insist upon holding and touching their newborn baby, even if hospital routine dictates that it be wrapped up and delivered to the nursery as soon as possible.

While it is true that the newborn has a tendency to chill (especially in a delivery room, which is maintained at a temperature comfortable for the staff), the infant who is dried well, then adequately covered and held by its mother has not been shown to have significantly more heat loss than the infant who is placed in a heated bassinet.[11]

The first hour or two after birth is a critical time for the mother–infant relationship. The infant, if it is not suffering the aftereffects of medications given to the mother during labor, is alert and responsive in a way that it will not be again for several days. Its eyes are open and can follow, and it attempts to focus on the mother's face if she is holding it. After the first hour or so it can no longer follow, and exhaustion sets in. The infant then becomes drowsy and is likely to be sleepy for 2 to 3 days.

Studies on the effects of increased early mother–child contact (some of which are ongoing) have shown interesting results in the area of mothering behavior (*e.g.*, increased fondling, holding in *en face* position) weeks after birth.[8] Other studies have shown measurable differences in children's IQ ratings up to 4 years after birth.[9] Although it is still early to draw definite conclusions, these results should certainly prompt a closer look at routine hospital practices that separate mother and child abruptly after birth and reestablish contact only after several hours. The infant needs the stroking and comforting of its mother in the first hours after birth, no less than the new mother needs the object of her concern to be responsive to her. To separate them arbitrarily at this crucial time is to do the family a grave disservice.

Integration has taken place when the fantasy child the couple had planned for is melded into the reality of the child that is here. Pointing out family characteristics of the newborn is a part of the process of acceptance and claiming. The childbirth educator can assist in this process by giving the prenatal couple a realistic idea of the newborn's appearance and behavior.

Integration of the newborn into the family constellation, be it a first child or later child, is a task that involves changes in all family relationships. It is several weeks before the confusion of the immediate postpartum quiets down and the couple begin to feel that they have some control over their lives agan. However, one study showed that by the end of 6 weeks most couples had made their adjustments, had "developed relatively ordered patterns of home life and baby care and seemed to be coping well with the realities of parenting."[5]

The Newborn

In describing the newborn to expectant parents, the childbirth educator should make as much use as possible of teaching aids. Many young persons have never seen a newborn and expect their child to resemble an infant who is 2 to 3 months old. If they are frightened by what appears to them to be abnormal, they will be hindered in their task of claiming, as they may fear making an emotional investment in this child. They need to be prepared for the immaturity of the newborn.

The instructor should begin by discussing the appearance of the newborn, including such frequently overlooked variations as moulding,

fontanelles, caput succedaneum, facial edema, **lanugo, vernix,** and the appearance of the skin (mottling, **cyanosis** of the extremities, **mongolian spots**). The relative size of the **genitalia** should be described. Parents should know that a female baby occasionally has a slight pink vaginal discharge, which is caused by the high level of hormones acquired from her mother and which subsides when the hormone level declines to that level normal for an infant in a few days. For the same reason, some infants may exhibit temporary breast engorgement and possibly secrete a few drops of what is known in old wives' tales as "witches' milk." This has usually passed by the eighth or ninth day. The instructor should also describe the appearance of the umbilical cord, both immediately and a few days later when it has dried and shriveled, scablike. It usually falls off by the end of the first week. Parents need to know that the only care required is to keep it clean and dry.

If the parents wish their male infant to be circumcised, it is usually done the day before discharge from the hospital, except in the case of a ritual **circumcision** on the eighth day for those of the Jewish faith. Occasionally the expectant parents in a prenatal class want to discuss the relative merits of circumcisions. Some feel that it should be done almost routinely on male infants for hygienic reasons; because, should it ever be necessary, it is a far more major operation in later life; or because other males in the family are circumcised. The only real medical indication is phimosis of the penis, which is relatively rare. Others feel that it should not be done unless clinically indicated because it is an unnecessary surgical procedure.

It is extremely important to mention the color of the newborn immediately after birth. The dramatic change from bluish to purple to bright pink is normal and wonderful to see, but it can terrify the new parents if they have not been forewarned. It can be explained in simple terms that, when the infant is moving down the birth canal, the cord is no longer supplying as much oxygen. As the oxygen level in the fetal blood falls, the carbon dioxide level rises, resulting in a bluish color. It is this buildup of carbon dioxide that stimulates the respiratory center in the brain and causes the infant to draw its first breath.

The fetus has an extra supply of hemoglobin, the oxygen-carrying component of the blood, to ensure an adequate oxygen supply while in the birth canal. This extra supply begins to break down after birth when its usefulness is past, resulting in physiological jaundice on about the third day.

To help the parents to begin thinking about the postnatal period, the instructor should initiate a discussion of the infant's needs. This can be managed very nicely by discussion techniques, with the leader only occasionally adding to the discussion. Content is not as important as making the parents aware that their baby is an individual with needs that he must learn to communicate. In the early weeks, parents and child are both learning to communicate in order to meet these needs.

The infant's needs include, of course, food and warmth, but also, and equally important, closeness and comfort, sucking and love. How his needs are met in the early weeks can have an effect on later socialization and learning. The parents do not need to fear they will spoil their newborn by picking him up and so forth, because his physical and emotional needs are inseparable. Love is shown by holding him close and secure while feeding, by talking, and by stroking him. As his parents learn to respond to his communication, the infant develops a basic trust that will color his attitudes throughout his life.

The parents also need to know that at times they will resent the relentless demands of the newborn. It should be brought out in class that this does not make them bad parents, because otherwise they may experience guilt about their natural feelings.

References

1. Antle K: Psychologic involvement in pregnancy by expectant father. JOGN 4(4):40-42, 1975
2. Audio Digest Foundation: Psychosomatic OB-GYN (tape). Obstet Gynecol 23(19), 1976
3. Edwards M: Communications: Dimensions in Childbirth Education. Copyright by the author, 1973
4. Eiger M, Olds S: THe Complete Book of Breastfeeding. New York, Workman Press, 1972
5. Fein R: The first weeks of fathering: The importance of choices and supports for new parents. Birth and the Family Journal 3:2, 1976
6. Heise J: Toward a better preparation for involved fatherhood. JOGN 4(5): 32-35, 1975
7. Hellman LM, Pritchard JA: Williams Obstetrics, 14th ed. New York, Appleton-Century-Crofts, 1971
8. Klaus M: Maternal attachment: The importance of the first post partum days. N Engl J Med 286:460, 1972
9. Klaus M: Presented at an Action for Newborns Conference, Columbus, Ohio, October 1974
10. Masters W, Johnson V: Human Sexual Response, pp 150-163. Boston, Little, Brown & Co, 1966
11. Phillips C: Neonatal heat loss in heated cribs vs mothers' arms. JOGN 3(6):11-15, 1974
12. Rozdilsky M, Banet B: What Now? A Handbook for Parents Post Partum. Copyright by the authors, 1972
13. Zalar M: Sexual counseling for pregnant couples. Matern Child Nurs J 1:176-181, 1976

10

Implementing the Prepared Childbirth Program

Organization of Classes

Classes may be designed for students at any phase of pregnancy, depending upon the resources and aims of the instructor or her employers as well as how early in pregnancy contact is established with the client group. Classes in psychoprophylaxis are basically a preparation for labor and delivery and should be given as close to term as possible when motivation runs high. If the instructor offers other information, classes may begin earlier in pregnancy with the preparation for labor and delivery saved for later classes. Conditioning is an essential element in **PPM** and, once techniques are learned, repetition in practice is needed.

Class sessions ordinarily last 1½ to 2 hours with a break in the middle. If the group is composed of women without their mates, the classes may be offered in the daytime, perhaps in conjunction with their office or clinic visit. If couples are attending together, the classes must usually be offered in the evening or on weekends to fit into the work schedules of the participants

Setting

The setting for the classes must have enough space for the women or couples to perform the exercise techniques being taught. The room should be well ventilated and as free from distractions as possible. The bathroom facilities should be nearby so that people can come and go without interrupting or calling attention to themselves.

For the discussion or content portion of the class, the group should be seated informally around a table, in a circle, or on the floor. If pillows are not available, the participants can be asked to bring two pillows to class with them.

Not every instructor is in a position to choose when or where she will teach, and classrooms may be far from ideal; however, the instructor must be alert to elements in the environment that may impede the interactive process of teaching and learning. There should be no physical barrier between the leader and her clients, because such barriers make the leader seem inaccessible. Examples of this kind of physical barrier include a uniform, which sets the instructor apart from those wearing street clothes. If the classroom is set up with a desk, podium, or table to stand or sit behind, the instructor can easily eliminate the barrier by standing or sitting on or in front of it. If many or most of the students are sitting on the floor, the instructor should get down to their level so that the dialogue that develops will flow laterally rather than up and down.

Fees

Class fees vary according to the contract the instructor has with her clients or her employers. If the instructor is hired by a hospital, the hospital often pays her a salary and the learners pay any fees directly to the hospital. In other cases the hospital provides the room, and the instructors get a percentage of each course fee. Either of these arrangements may also be used when a physician or group of physicians offer classes in their office.

Sometimes a childbirth education association, made up either of instructors alone or of professional and parent members, is formed. The association may be in a position to subsidize the instructor's salary through fund-raising events such as film showings. The association may also offer classes on subjects other than childbirth preparation, such as parenting and breast-feeding, or support other groups that do offer these classes. Usually, though not always, the sponsoring agency maintains control by handling the registration and fees.

Sometimes individual childbirth instructors set up a private practice. They may offer classes in their homes or in a local "Y," church, or other community facility. In this instance the instructor is paid by her clients.

The amount of the fee depends upon the custom and resources of the community and whether or not the instructor is subsidized by a sponsoring agency. Hospitals may wish to offer the course free as a community service or at a minimal fee only. The professional childbirth educator who wants to go into private practice will have to explore the prices paid in her community to establish a fair fee for her professional services. (As a very broad rule of thumb, it can be said that the fee for a childbirth preparation course is usually slightly less than 10% of the going obstetric fee in the same area.)

If their physician recommends that they attend classes as a part of their prenatal care, expectant parents should be informed that the fee may be a tax deductible medical expense. Their payment should be made out to Jane Doe, RN, and receipts should be given.

If couples who cannot afford to pay the usual fee apply for classes, many instructors are willing to try to work out a mutually satisfactory arrangement, especially if no other resource is available to these couples.

Some agencies offer the courses without charge, although many feel that even a minimal investment as a registration fee increases the probability of faithful practice and attendance and thus enhances the value of the program.

Class Size

If the childbirth educator were offering mere training for childbirth, the class could be any size. However, since she should get to know her clients well enough to have some idea of their individual needs, she should limit the size of the class. The childbirth educator who is working under the auspices of a hospital may not have complete control over the class size, but she should try to keep the instructor–student ratio down to around 1:15 individuals, or about 1:8-10 couples. In larger groups individuals may hesitate to speak up and make their needs known.[1,2]

Some instructors have worked around this problem by having helpers work with individuals during exercise sessions. This is an improvement but still fails to meet the need for each person to participate in his or her own learning. It is all too easy in this setting to go back to the authoritarian lecture style, in which case learner needs will not be met.

Recruitment

The first task of recruitment is to make potential clients aware that classes are available. Hospitals may send out brochures or announcements, or they may display posters prominently. Organized childbirth groups may do the same, but the individual who is offering classes may be discouraged from publicizing them in these ways. There is a feeling among professionals that individuals should not advertise their services. The genesis of this attitude seems to be the split between what is perceived as "professional" and what may be termed "mercantile." This is all very well if you have an institution to do the advertising for you, but the educator who wants to go into private practice, a nontraditional role for nurses, must come to grips with the reality of the situation. There is no real barrier to announcing the program by the same means available to institutions and other groups. Posters in supermarkets or community centers fall within this framework. A community bulletin board might be another good location for an annoucement.

Overtures may be made to the physicians who do the deliveries in the community. Many may misunderstand what is taught in class, or they may have had a previous bad experience and hestitate to recommend classes. A brochure or letter explaining the overall objectives of the course may be the initial contact, followed by a phone call. Professional cards may be included wth the introductory letter if desired (see Fig. 1–1).

The childbirth educator might also contact the local hospital and find out if they will support the classes. Since the instructor must work closely with the labor room staff to assure continuity of care for her students, enlisting the support of the obstetric supervisor when trying to establish a childbirth preparation program is the first step in the direction of mutual cooperation. If the hospital is not ready to sponsor the classes, the instructor can ask how she can best prepare her students for the hospital experience, and what the hospital staff would like the laboring couples to know. Communications between the hospital and the childbirth educator is important if the students are to be given a realistic and valid preparation. Communication is enhanced if the instructor asks for feedback. Did the hospital staff feel that the couples were well prepared? What suggestions can they make to improve the preparation?

Other ways to bring the availability of classes to the attention of potential clients might be to write an article on the need for childbirth preparation for the local newspaper or to have a film showing by renting one or more of the childbirth films currently available for a modest rental fee.

Lower Socioeconomic Clients

Unlike the motivated middle-class expectant parents who are eager to participate in the birth of their child and who can see the advantages of preparation, the poor or lower socioeconomic clients do not give a high priority to childbirth preparation. First, a distinction must be made between the temporarily poor (*e.g.*, student couples) who do not currently have resources but who are more closely aligned to the middle-class couple in terms of values, and the chronically deprived lower class. (The educator must beware of making assumptions about individuals, however.) These multiproblem families share disadvantages such as poverty, poor living conditions, little education, and, most significantly perhaps, little control over their lives or the direction of the future.

Because the multiplicity of their problems means there is little reward for effort, many poor people have an aversion to making plans for the future. Setting goals even for self-help is primarily a middle-class attribute. People with few choices have little practice in making decisions and may become apathetic. In addition, the poor may see a childbirth class as just one more attempt to impose middle-class values on them and may feel that it is unrealistic for their situation.

Again, because the poor have so few options, they do not value independence; dependence upon others (individuals or institutions) is seen as desirable. If they do decide to attend class, they may need help in arranging for transportation or baby-sitting.

The instructor cannot expect these clients to come out of their own environment to attend classes. She must go to them and must be ready to offer assistance and suggestions to make class attendance less problematical (*e.g.*, the class might be held in their clinic, community center, church, or "Y"). The instructor can try to make community leaders see the value of a childbirth program and enlist their aid. Often these leaders make suggestions for a location or recruitment. In order to involve a community in meeting its own needs, the educator must be aware of and use its systems.

Obviously, in a situation where the instructor is more interested in giving the classes than her clients may be in attending them, funding for the program must come from other resources. Funds may come from a hospital or public health agency that wishes to offer community outreach programs or from a social service or community agency that can see the value of childbirth preparation.

In this situation it is appropriate to distribute simple flyers, bilingual where applicable, and to display posters in supermarkets, storefronts, and so forth. News releases in popular papers or announcements on local radio or TV programs may also be useful. Public service announcements may be made by radio stations without charge for noncommercial programs.[4] If possible, the childbirth educator should get to know the target commuity by walking around, going to community meetings, and shopping in the area. She should learn about the available transportation and the existing conditions of the area.

Meeting the Needs of the Group

Each group is different just as each instructor is unique in the ways she interacts with the group. Although teachers of PPM may have similar general objectives for the course, the order of presentation and emphasis may differ. The teacher must adapt her knowledge and skills to the learning needs of her particular students. In planning an educational program, the same steps are followed as in the nursing process.*

Assessment

Learner needs are assessed by collecting data from observation and from nonverbal as well as verbal communication. The teacher assesses the attitudes of her students and asks for active participation from them in identifying their needs. She then uses the information they supply about their needs plus her own specialized knowledge of the physical and psychological needs of the childbearing cycle to decide what her approach

---

* Based on *The Nursing Process*, a paper from the Committee on Practice. Presented at The Nurses Association of the American College of Obstetricians and Gynecologists (ACOG), Chicago, April, 1976

should be for this particular group. This step is valid for the program as a whole as well as for particular topics.

Planning

After assessing the learners' needs in relation to her own goals, the instructor plans for this particular group, that is, tailors her program to fit their needs. For example, highly educated groups might feel uneasy with a discussion approach. Being accustomed to a more structured classroom situation, these students often have difficulty in seeing the value of seemingly contentless discussion; they need to learn how to use the group. Explanations must be detailed and clear for this type of group. They want facts and may have more difficulty in talking about feelings. The instructor in this group must be aware of their need for more content and at the same time work to make the coming childbirth experience seem more real in terms of the emotions surrounding it.

Implementation

Implementation is following through on the plan for teaching or teaching intervention as decided in the assessment and planning phases.

Evaluation

Evaluation is an esential component for dynamic group sessions. Without evaluation, classes become static and rigid in approach. Evaluation may be accomplished by asking for feedback from students (during classes and postpartum) and from others on the health care team.

Self-evaluation is also important. The instructor must be constantly alert to verbal and nonverbal cues from her group that tell her when she is not getting across or when the group feels good about something. Only by taking the trouble to reflect on and evaluate her teaching can the childbirth educator sharpen her skills to enhance the learning process for her students.

For example, if Sally Smith asks about episiotomies by demanding, "Do they really rip you down there?", the instructor *assesses* by realizing that there is a great deal of anxiety and perhaps misconception about episiotomies. She may ask the class what they have heard about episiotomies. She *plans* teaching intervention. She *implements* her plan by explaining in more detail than usual how episiotomies are done, why many obstetricians feel that it is advantageous to do an episiotomy, and how the mother herself can reduce postpartum pain. Finally, she *evaluates* her teaching by asking for feedback and discussion in a subsequent class. She might also ask Sally Smith herself if her stitches are bothering her in her postpartum follow-up.

Learning

Facilitating Learning

The skill and personality of the leader has a great deal of influence on whether or not the childbirth class truly prepares expectant parents for birth or simply trains them. Rogers describes the attributes desirable in a teacher.[3] Learning is facilitated when the teacher is openly aware of the person she is. She must be aware of her own attitudes and accept her own feelings without imposing them upon the group. At the same time the instructor must understand the student as he or she is and emphathize with his or her feelings. Her acceptance of any or all feelings expressed in the group (unconditional positive regard) shows respect for each student as a person and not just as another group member.

Other ways to communicate respect and caring to people in the group is to establish eye contact when a student is speaking and to learn each student's name. It is not always easy to learn names in groups of any size, but it is well worth the trouble if it can be managed. One strategy in remembering people is to repeat their names as they introduce themselves and then use every opportunity to say the names again. For example, if Maria Lopez has introduced herself and later wants to ask a question, the instructor can take the opportunity to recognize her by name: "Yes, Maria?", instead of just "Yes?" This reinforces the association between the name and the face. After the first class session, the instructor can sit down with the registration cards and go through each one, trying to place the name with the face and to recall any significant detail to fix it in her mind. Another review of the cards before the next session is usually sufficient. To be positive, the instructor might greet the students by name as they come in. This can facilitate learning by giving each participant the feeling that the leader is interested in him or her personally.

The learning process is also enhanced if the learner experiences success. For this reason the leader not only reinforces the woman's ability herself, but teaches the coach to make positive remarks and to validate what the woman is doing right before correcting what she is doing wrong.

Barriers to Learning

Learning is hindered if the couple feel uncomfortable in their surroundings or anxious about either themselves or class content. Anxiety unrelated to the class may interfere with learning as well; for example, if the husband has lost his job, if exams are coming up at school, or if they had an argument just before coming to class, they may well be preoccupied. Physical discomfort also interferes with learning, and the leader must be alert to subtle clues if someone hesitates to ask if a window could be opened or closed, and so forth.

Some couples play manipulative games with each other or with the instructor. Occasionally the coach is coercing his wife into coming to class because he wants to be present for the birth, although she does not want to be awake. Other times the couple may offer all kinds of excuses why they cannot find time to practice together when the real reason may be a hesitance to involve themselves because of anxiety or disinterest.

Apparent disinterest may very well mask hidden anxiety and denial. People with poor self-images, who feel they cannot succeed or take advantage of opportunities, may find it difficult to learn.

Group Process

A group may be defined as a collection of people who come together to work on common needs or tasks. The childbirth class is a group of expectant parents who come together to work on childbirth and early parenting. The leader or sponsoring agency offers a setting that is hospitable to these tasks.

Terms borrowed from the social worker may be used to explain the process that evolves with each group meeting as well as with the overall development of the group itself.

The first phase in group process is the *tuning-in phase*. This is the initial interaction between students and leader in the group setting, the time when each is feeling out the surroundings. Receptive to veiled communication, the instructor looks for cues and listens for themes and attitudes. For example, if most are in casual attire and one coach chooses to keep his jacket and tie on, he may not wish to identify himself as a part of the group. The places that students choose to sit may be another kind of communication. Couples who choose to sit far from the instructor may be fearful of becoming too involved right away. Those who choose to sit apart from each other may disagree about coming to class. The students are looking for cues from the leader at the same time. Does she make an effort to put them at ease? If she busies herself with her papers and ignores them as they enter, they may get the message that she does not wish to involve herself personally with them.

The second phase may be termed the *contractual phase*. In this phase, introductions are made and interaction begins. The leader tells the group who she is, generally what her background is, and what to expect from her. She then asks each member of the class to introduce himself or herself. Together the group and the instructor explore the contract (the merging of the participants' tasks and the instructor's tasks). The instructor should be aware of any hidden agendas (ulterior motives), either from the couples or from her employers. For example, does the leader see herself as the agent of the couples? Or is she employed by a hospital to prepare the parents to cooperate with the hospital? This may make a difference in the way things are presented.

The third phase in the process is the *work period*. That is the time when the group is getting on with the tasks in the contract. The instructor should recognize when work is being done and reinforce this behavior with positive comments. When it is being evaded, her reminder that the techniques will not be as predictable or effective without practice may help to remotivate the couple.

The final phase in group process is the *transition and ending phase*. The conclusion of the class or course, when the work period is finished, may be a difficult time in the group because of feelings of separation, but the leader should focus on the next step. She can make a brief summary of the work accomplished and give an overview of the next meeting. If it is the final meeting of the course, the leader can suggest that the group members keep in touch with each other as well as with her. Sometimes a postpartum meeting can be arranged to continue group support.

These phases in group process occur in each class and also in the course as a whole. The class outline at the close of Chapter 1 (Table 1-1) shows the tuning-in phase in the initial interactions between the instructor and students. Each is sounding the other out as they state their reasons for being there. In a sense, the entire first class is devoted to the tuning-in and contractual phases. Although learning takes place when the theory of PPM and the labor overview are given, these topics also explain and clarify the instructor's plan to her students. In the life of the group, then, the first class is mainly tuning in and contractual even though the work period begins with the presentation of physical fitness exercises and the controlled relaxation preparatory exercise. The middle block of classes may be viewed as the work period; labor and delivery are covered in detail, and the various appropriate techniques are learned and practiced.

At the final class the students are usually very much aware of the coming separation. The instructor stresses her own continuing interest and concern and that of the other group members.

References

1. Auerbach A: Parents Learn Through Discussion, p 157. New York, John Wiley & Sons, 1968
2. Auerbach A: Preparation for Parenthood Through Group Discussion. New Brunswick, NJ, Johnson & Johnson, 1976
3. Rogers C: On Becoming a Person. Boston, Houghton Mifflin, 1961
4. Stein T: Establishing prenatal classes in a small community. Journal of Obstetrics, Gynecology, and Neonatal Nursing 2:44–47, 1973

11

Program Development

The First Class

Tuning In

The childbirth educator faced with a new class must first find out what attitudes and impressions of labor her students have. Perhaps the most direct approach is simply to ask each individual why he or she decided to come to class. What do they think the program can or should do for them? This indicates respect for each individual, gives the instructor an idea of what the person thinks, and helps to create bonds between class members as they hear their own concerns reflected in the words of others. By correcting obvious misinformation and by validating the reality of each member's feelings, the mood of acceptance is set as the class moves from the tuning-in period into the contractual phase.

Setting the Contract

It is important at this point to establish clearly the goals of the program as well as its limitations. It is unfair to the student and the instructor, for example, to let the student believe that coming to the course assures her of an effortless and painless birth. One can never promise an easy birth, let alone a painless one. Realistically, the childbirth educator can offer only the tools to cope with the labor that occurs. If the expectations of the instructor and students are not established at the beginning of the course, the progress of the work that can be accomplished by the program is hampered.

Programs that are based entirely upon discussion techniques use the contractual phase of the first class to gather the agenda for the course. The expectant parents express the concerns that are most important to them, and the curriculum is developed upon this base. Proponents of this approach feel that in this way the program more nearly fulfills the needs of the specific participants of a group.[2]

Unlike the straight discussion approach to childbirth education, preparation for birth by PPM requires a more directive approach. Since psychoprophylaxis depends on conditioning, repetition and reinforcement are essential if the conditioning process is to take place. There are certain essential elements that the leader *must* give the class members (*e.g.*, controlled relaxation and respiratory techniques for labor). This is a part of the contract. Little time, therefore, is spent in agenda gathering.

Expectant parents have a multitude of questions. Some are overt, waiting only to be asked. Others are less obvious—half-hidden fears and myths that are a part of a student's cultural heritage. The student may accept these myths unquestioningly or may be afraid to ask about them for fear of appearing foolish. This is an important consideration for the instructor. She would like to help the students to voice their concerns, but they may hesitate for fear of exposing themselves to ridicule. One approach to this dilemma is the use of the "some people believe. . ." or "has anyone ever told you . . ." tactic, then asking what other things the students have heard. In this manner, old wives' tales can be brought out into the open for discussion without forcing people to admit that they half-believed them to be true.

This fear of exposure may be observed when questions are prefaced by such statements as "this may be a stupid question" or even "my mother-in-law says . . ." as a protective mechanism. The sensitive teacher knows that, although the desire to know was stronger than the fear of seeming ignorant in this case, the way in which she accepts the first question determines if the class will be willing to discuss anxieties or not. The instructor should always validate what the speaker is feeling before going on to explain or correct. Certainly she does not leave her group with misinformation; however, in framing her reply, she ensures that she reinforces the listeners' desire to learn by accepting their concerns.

In deciding what information to present, the teacher should keep in mind that, using words as a therapeutic tool, she is constantly working to strengthen students' coping mechanisms. Teaching aids such as charts, graphs, slides, and a knitted uterus are all valuable adjuncts. These need not be expensive; many are available for very little or may be made by the instructor herself (see Appendix C).

Equally important, care must be taken to use language that may be easily grasped by the group. It is helpful to use everyday events as examples because new learning can be enhanced if the learner can relate it to something he or she already knows. For example, comparing the physical conditioning process of an athlete in preparation for an athletic event with preparation for the physical event of birth makes good common sense and reinforces the need for preparation and for discipline in practice.

It is helpful if the first class includes an overview of the entire course, including objectives. In the discussion-type class this is taken care of by the gathering of the agenda. In the more structured class it gives an idea of the material to be included and helps the couple to organize their thoughts about labor, birth, and their respective roles in the process.

The Work Period

Often the childbirth instructor may ask the group members what they have heard or read to try to assess how much information the group already has and where she may profitably begin. Some instructors prefer to suggest reading to be done prior to class attendance to provide a learning baseline.

The Coach

Since the labor coach has a definite role in the PPM approach, care must be taken at the outset to include him and explain his importance. Very few expectant fathers who come to the first class have any clear idea of what it is they will be expected to do. Understandably, a fair percentage of these prospective labor coaches hesitate to involve themselves. The woman has no choice—it is she who gives birth to the baby—but the father can choose whether to involve himself or not. External pressures such as bloody depictions of childbirth on film and television with the woman out of control and in agony, the half-joking derision of his peers who talk about "women's work" and how they would never want to be there, and a lack of accurate information combine to heighten his feeling of helplessness. If he is fearful about what he will witness or how he himself will perform, he may prefer to withdraw.

Often the expectant father does not want to expose these feelings. But if they can be brought out into the open and talked about, it helps to set the tone of acceptance. The instructor can initiate this discussion by remarking that many (or most) men may have come to class primarily because their wives dragged them there. This generally brings a rueful laugh and sidelong glances between husband and wife.

If the childbirth teacher can then incite the coach's interest by helping him to see how rewarding his involvement will be to himself as well as to his wife and child, she will have enlisted the aid of a most stalwart provider of moral support.

The coach must know exactly what his role entails. During the preparatory period he is responsible for helping his wife to learn and perform the various techniques that she may expect to employ during labor. Therefore, he must learn what she is expected to do and how she looks when she is performing correctly. He also must know what problems may develop and how he can best help her to overcome them. To fulfill this task he must learn the techniques himself, at least well enough to recognize difficulties when they occur, by participating in regular disciplined practice periods. He should also recognize the subtle difference between helping her to achieve and directing her to perform, the latter implying the imposition of his will upon her. The use of such words as "coach" as opposed to "direct" helps to make this distinction clear.

The Mother

The mother too must accept responsibility. It is not enough to say that she will produce the infant. She too must accept the disciplines of practice to learn the various techniques. She must communicate openly with the physician or midwife and the childbirth educator to learn the answers to her questions. Only in this way can the childbirth team begin to function as a unit. In labor she is responsible for her own behavior, although she can expect the support and assistance of the labor coach, the labor room nurse, and the physician or midwife.

The Facts

Having set the tone by clarifying what will be expected of each member of the childbirth team and having shown herself open to questions and ideas, the instructor is ready to move on in the work period by providing facts relevant to current concerns.

The first task may be to explain how PPM works and how it relates to comfort and pain in labor. It is essential that each group member have a grasp of the concept of "what makes it work" if they are to apply the principles of conditioning, concentration, and discipline in practice and application. The explanation must be as clear and uncomplicated as possible, and ample time must be allotted for questions.

After the explanation, the instructor can ask for feedback, perhaps asking the group to contribute examples of how the principles work from their own lives. The fact that concentrating on a movie blocks out the perception of a headache would be one example. One young expectant father brought up the following example of conditioning leading to a predictable response. It seems that he had been training in the paratroopers several years before and he, like most of his classmates, was terrified of making the first real jump. An hour before the first jump was scheduled, the drill master had them all line up on a low bench and ordered them to jump off the bench each time they heard the command, "One, two, three, jump!" He then spent a full hour having them jump to the verbal command, climb onto the bench and jump again. The process must have been repeated about 50 times. Following this episode, they were taken up for the first jump, and they all responded automatically when their leader used the verbal cue, "One, two, three, jump!"

Once the principles of PPM are accepted and there has been enough free-flowing discussion for the leader to feel sure they have been understood, she can move on to present an overview of labor and delivery. How much information is included depends upon the needs of the group and the time available. If ample time is available, it may be a good idea to begin by reviewing body changes during pregnancy, especially if the group has not had the benefit of meeting together in early pregnancy. If time is not available, then the emphasis may be on the upcoming labor and delivery, because this is where most concerns are centered in the final weeks. Even if the instructor feels that time is limited, she must be prepared to include information on body changes if questions arise.

Group members are usually eager to begin preparing for labor and delivery. As the work period of the first class nears its end, physical fitness exercises may be introduced in the framework or helping the body to be in the best possible physical condition for the physical stresses of labor. Explanations can be given about the need for improved circulation and muscle tone for labor as well as for increased comfort in the prenatal period. This can be related to what has already been said about the childbearing continuum, with the body already preparing itself for the changes that will take place during labor.

To pull in the coach in the first class and to begin the interpersonal interaction between coach and parturient, the preparatory exercise for controlled relaxation should be included (Appendix A). If the couple work on achieving the feeling of total relaxation in the first week, they will be ready to move on to relaxing under stress by the next meeting.

Transition and Ending

As the class nears its end, the instructor should draw together all the bits and pieces of information that have been covered in the work period. She may do this easily by summarizing what was discussed and relating topics that were covered near the end to principles that were discussed earlier (*e.g.*, relating the use of precise verbal cues and the need to practice controlled relaxation faithfully to the principles of conditioning, concentration, and discipline). She may finish by reminding them briefly what the focus of the next meeting will be.

The childbirth educator is not quite finished when the class period ends. It will be profitable if she spends some time reflecting upon how the class went. She should ask herself is she accomplished everything she hoped to accomplish in the session. If not, she can plan to bring up areas that may not have been covered fully or that may not have been clearly understood in the following session.

Second and Third Classes

Each class in the series should begin with a review of what was covered in the previous class. The leader might begin by asking the group if they have any questions on the previous discussion. She needs to be comfortable with silence while she awaits her reply, as some students hesitate to be the first to raise a question. If no one asks a question, she might summarize briefly, then move on into the work period by reviewing the physical fitness and controlled relaxation preparatory exercises.

As the couples do the exercises, the instructor can assess their skill, correct problems, and generally reinforce their strengths. In the controlled relaxation exercise, she can begin to see how the couple interact with each other. The coaching role becomes clearer as the coach learns how to give verbal and tactile cues and the woman learns how to respond appropriately.

Once the exercises that were included in the previous session have been reviewed, it is time to build on them. Physical fitness exercises that were not included in the first session and the practice exercise in controlled relaxation may be added (Appendix A). The couple has had a week to practice the preparatory exercise demonstrated in the previous class. By now they should have a good awareness of tension and relaxation.

Once this awareness has been achieved, they are already to move on to the problem of relaxing the body when one muscle area is tensed (as the uterus will be in labor). The woman is instructed to contract, for example, her right arm. After tightening this area, she concentrates upon relaxing the rest of her body. The coach looks for visual and tactile clues that tell him tension is present. He uses what he has learned in the previous week about verbal cues and stroking to signal its release. Finally, when he is satisfied that the rest of the body is relaxed, he strokes the tensed arm and asks her to "relax your right arm." This practice drill is repeated using other body areas or perhaps having the woman tense more than one area at a time as she becomes more proficient. The coach may need to be reminded to keep his emphasis always on the relaxation aspects.

The overall focus for the second class might be on the beginning of labor, early labor, and early active labor. By the end of the third session most instructors have pretty well covered the first stage of labor, including the work being accomplished, the woman's changing mood, the coaching role, the characteristics of the contractions and variations. It is appropriate to include information about medications that might be used in the first stage, as well as induction or stimulation of labor.

Certainly any questions that come up should be discussed. Although discussion techniques make it difficult to use any predecided order of presentation, a careful review of what was just covered at the end of each class session makes it easy to follow up in the next. Taking care of questions as they arise shows respect for the learners' concerns and is far more important than following an outline, even if the childbirth educator is not able to present every single fact to each and every class.

Respiratory techniques for labor are also presented one step at a time. The various techniques are divided into two basic breathing techniques for easy learner acceptance. After the students have become comfortable with the basic techniques, the breathing progression as it applies to labor is easy to assimilate because it builds upon skills they already have.

Fourth and Fifth Classes

After the first stage of labor has been fairly well covered, the class is ready to learn about the second and third stages. Barriers to acceptance include anxiety about performance, body image, and separation (*i.e.*, loss of pregnant state). Careful explanation with the use of pictures and therapeutic language helps to dispel fears. A series such as *Birth Atlas*, which depicts the internal and external rotations as the infant negotiates the pelvis, can be reassuring.* (How graphic this should be depends upon the group.) Descriptions of the work, the mood of the mother, and the characteristics of the contractions and how they feel to the mother help to structure expectation. Although the instructor cannot promise a peak experience, she can promise that the second stage will be better than the transition phase. Most important, she can excite the couples about working to see their child born and to hear its first cry.

Continuing to teach complicated exercises one step at a time, the instructor teaches the preparatory exercise for expulsion, then labor room pushing. After each step is explained, time must be allotted to repeat important points and ask for feedback from each learner before adding the next step.

Rather than close the class with something entirely new, the instructor may remind the group of the need to rest and return to complete relaxation between contractions. This can be reinforced by finishing with controlled relaxation, which should be practiced using the position the woman will be in between contractions (propped up at about a 35° angle).

By the close of the fifth session there are no new techniques to add and the whole pattern of labor and delivery can be put together. This can be accomplished in several ways that reinforce knowledge the couples already have. The instructor may choose to use a role-playing situation, directing an imaginary labor from start to finish. She can include as much review as necessary by asking the couples to act out how they would respond if it were an actual labor. Instead of or in addition to role playing, slides or a movie of childbirth may be used. Since the expectant parents are by now quite knowledgeable about what to look for, seeing other couples going through labor with the use of techniques that they too have learned is reassuring. Any particular points the leader wants to make can be made during slide showings, but slides should precede a film so that the parents can involve themselves in the film without interruption. Variations, such as cesarean birth, can be included here. Time should be allotted afterward to allow for discussion.

Sixth Class

For many this is the final session in a prenatal series. Although some work may still be accomplished, the instructor should not introduce too much new material because feelings about separation may interfere with integration. If the group was able to complete its work on the stages of labor, the sixth session may profitably be devoted to learning about the

---

Birth Atlas is published by Maternity Center Association. (See Appendix C for address.)

postpartum and new parenting experience. Because of their overriding concern with labor and delivery, the couples may find it difficult to accept the reality of the postpartum period. Emphasizing the mutuality of postpartum stresses will help them cope with these stresses when they actually occur, however little they seem to accept them before the birth. Explaining some of the stresses that each person undergoes while reemphasizing to the couple the importance of communicating their feelings to each other is also helpful.

The discussion may also focus on the newborn, if the appearance and behavior of the newborn infant has not been covered earlier. Discussion techniques can be supplemented by appropriate teaching aids such as the pamphlets available from Ross Laboratories or Mead Johnson (see Resource List, Appendix C).

If new parents from a previous class can come to this session with their new baby, this can be a profitable experience for all. They can relate what labor was really like for them and talk about postpartum adjustments. They also have the advantage of being able to show off the reason for all the preparation, and the expectant parents can observe for themselves what a tiny infant looks like.

Classes With Special Needs

Some classes beg further attention because they may require a modified approach. These include low-income groups, unwed expectant mothers, and teenagers. Classes for these special groups are usually sponsored by the health care facility that will be delivering the women. In the case of school-aged expectant mothers, classes may be offered through the school system in an effort to help these youngsters stay in school. Childbirth preparation is most often a part of a coordinated plan involving educational, health, and social service agencies.

Women who do not have a coach may hesitate to involve themselves in classes made up of couples. Although some highly motivated single women do choose to join a regular group, these are usually women who have a good sense of self-esteem and do not feel too threatened by the fact that all the other participants are in pairs. Others may prefer to attend groups made up of women who share their special problems.

Some of these women do not take advantage of classes that are offered because they believe women cannot "use natural childbirth" without a coach. Their low self-esteem may cause them to believe that they are incapable of achieving anything worthwhile, or they may simply be unable to see how preparation could be relevant to their individual needs.

People learn best when they are offered what they desire to learn. They cannot learn what is unacceptable to them or what they see as irrelevant. For this reason, a guided discussion approach is probably best for these special-need groups. An approach based upon the fact that learning these exercises and techniques helps the woman to feel better, experience a more comfortable labor, and recover faster after the baby is born is a practical way to broach the subject. They will become motivated if they can see how they will be able to use what they learn.

Teen-aged Expectant Mothers

The birth that is experienced by the very young woman may have far-reaching effects upon her future sexual adjustments or later birth experiences. If the childbirth educator can help her to have a reasonably good experience, one that she can recall with a sense of accomplishment, it may enhance her self-esteem and make later adjustments smoother. If she does not have the support of the baby's father, the mutuality of shared concerns of the group can reduce the sense of isolation so commonly seen in women alone.

The teenaged expectant mother is still struggling with the problem of identity. She does not yet have a clear idea of who she is as a person, much less as a mother. Reflections from the peer group are immensely important to the teen-ager in defining who she is, yet the pregnancy often means increasing isolation from those very friends. They simply do not have the same problems.

Often the teenaged expectant mother's concern is focused primarily on herself—how she feels or how she will manage her problems—rather than on the coming infant. Having not yet achieved a sense of her own identity, it is difficult for her to form an internalized image of the baby as an individual. Anxiety may be centered around her changing body and whether she will be permanently marked by stretch marks and scars.

Too often her care is fragmented or not formulated with her individual needs in mind. For example, she may be given information about proper diet and its importance for her growing baby with no regard for her own likes and dislikes. In addition, she may not be able to afford to change her eating patterns to meet the requirements. Unless these problems are resolved, it is unlikely that she will make the effort to change her eating habits.[1]

Close communication between all members of the health care team, including the expectant mother, is essential if a care plan is to be worked out that the parturient can realistically be expected to follow.[3] The childbirth instructor is in a position to reinforce the roles of other team members only if she is aware of the overall care plan. This knowledge provides the continuity that is necessary if the woman is to learn to trust the system and those who will care for her.

Unwed Expectant Mothers

The unwed mother who does not have a significant caring person in her life to give her support shares some of the same problems faced by the teenager. (Unwed expectant mothers who have a stable relationship with the expectant fathers are not included here, because these expectant parents fall into the category of couples regardless of their legal status.) She may or may not have matured enough to have a secure sense of self-identity, but she is often finished with the very basic schooling that pregnancy interrupts in the case of the teenager. She may even have had the opportunity to develop a self-image on the basis of her professional life.

On the other hand, unwed and teenaged expectant mothers share the problem of the baby's future. If the infant is not to be given up for adoption, plans must be made for its support and care (if the mother must return to her job). Group discussions often center around plans for day care or the future, because these women are generally more able to plan for the future than their teen-aged counterparts. As with the teenager, however, even these plans for the baby may have more to do with how the mother herself will cope with the infant. The unwed mother may see herself more as a woman with a problem than as a mother with a baby. If she is planning to give the baby up for adoption, she may ask about the possibility of abnormality because she knows that infants with problems are often hard to place. A useful approach to this type of question ("Will my baby be all right?") might be to emphasize that by eating a healthful diet, by getting good prenatal care, and by learning to help herself so that a minimum of medication is needed in labor, the woman is giving her child the best possible start in life. This idea may help mothers who may never be able to give this infant anything else.

Teaching the Woman Without a Coach

Women alone, that is, women who will give birth without the assistance of a supportive coach, will need to be highly motivated to learn and use the disciplines of psychoprophylaxis effectively for labor. In classes for couples, the instructor works to strengthen interdependence between expectant parents. When the woman will not be able to rely upon some significant caring person from her environment to coach her, she must be prepared from the beginning to work alone.

The emphasis in these classes should be on the woman's ability to help herself. Many women do come to class, prepare themselves, and manage very well in labor. It is more difficult for a woman to prepare herself than to prepare with the help and encouragement of someone else, but it can be done. If the woman expects to be alone in labor and delivery, she should prepare with that in mind.

From the start with controlled relaxation, she must take over the monitoring task of the coach. She must learn to recognize tension in herself and to cue its release. In the preparatory exercise she can run through a mental checklist more or less as the instructor does in class (see Appendix A). Beginning with the feet and alternately tightening and releasing toes, heels, ankles, legs, thighs, hips, buttocks, perineum, and so forth, she should mentally say the words "tighten" (or contract) and "release" (or relax), timing the relaxation to conincide with the exhalation. After she has consciously released each muscle group, she should try to relax it a bit more, then still more. The instructor can say, "Learn to know your body. How does it *feel* when it is tense? How does it *feel* when it is relaxed? The more *relaxed* you are, the more *comfortable* and less tired you will be. *Think* about letting go; really make you mind *concentrate* on being relaxed." The preparatory exercise ends when she takes another deep signal breath and releases all her voluntary muscles.

For the practice exercise in controlled relaxation under stress, the instructor asks the woman to contract one group of voluntary muscles while she concentrates on relaxing all other muscle groups. The drill is the same as the one used by the woman with a coach except that the woman alone uses her own mental cues rather than the verbal cues of a coach. She focuses first on tightening the target area, then on completely relaxing all the other areas. She must go through a mental checklist just as the coach would go through a visual and tactile checklist. She must ask herself, "Are my thighs relaxed? perineum? buttocks?" and so forth, and with each exhalation she must try to relax each area a little more. After she is satisfied, she releases the target area, takes another deep signal breath, and relaxes completely as she exhales. This same procedure can be followed with areas of the back, although it is difficult to detect tension in these areas. This important exercise should be reviewed in class at each meeting, with the teacher reinforcing the woman's efforts and abilities each time.

The same procedure is followed in the teaching of respiratory and expulsion techniques. The woman must be told the coaching points and be helped to integrate them. She should be reminded to use the appropriate cue words to condition a predictable response. At first she may practice in front of a mirror if this is helpful, but she should be encouraged to learn the feeling of correct technique rather than to depend upon the mirror for feedback.

Continuity of care is especially important for the woman who will not bring anyone with her into the labor room. The hospital staff might be alerted in advance if the parturient will need extra coaching. It is also important for the instructor to get in touch with her student postpartum to find out how things went and to offer constructive suggestions and support where appropriate.

Low-Income Groups

Unlike the unwed mother, the low-income woman may have an expectant father available for support, but too often the multiple problems with which they must live do not allow for his participation. Classes for this group are usually held at the community clinic during the day when the husband may be at work, or he may need to stay home to care for other children. Also, the additional carfare required for the father to come to classes may be a burden on the low-income family. Whatever the reason, clinic classes are often composed primarily of expectant mothers.

Because of the multiplicity of problems and because those outside of the situation cannot really understand what it is like to live in poverty, a discussion approach comes much closer to meeting the needs of the group than a formal lecture. It is a mistake for the professional to decide what is needed and attempt to meet that projected need. The exercise portion is the only portion of the classes that does not lend itself well to a discussion approach.

Discipline in practice is just as important for this group if responses are to be predictable for labor, but the instructor may not be successful in engendering the desire to use discipline in practice. The other needs of this group are so great that discipline may be an unrealistic expectation. In this case, the "try this, it may help you" approach may be more appropriate.

If the group is to begin to regard preparation for childbirth as realistic for them, the instructor must acknowledge that preparation for childbirth is not the main problem and that diligence in practice will not change their life situations. The problem is poverty itself. After the instructor recognizes this overriding fact, she can then begin to work on a problem that she *can* do something about: improving the birth experience.

Because low-income groups often suffer from low self-esteem as well as low social esteem, they have a great deal to gain from joining a group besides learning basic facts about childbirth. The unconditional positive regard and respect shown each individual in the group by the leader, as well as the mutual support of the group members, reinforces their self-images and in turn enhances their potential for learning.

If the classes are offered in the clinic setting, the childbirth educator may not even be able to take the group into a separate room for meetings. It may be necessary to begin with bench conferences on a one-to-one basis. Much teaching can be done this way, but the mutuality of the group interchange is lost. If the instructor is taking advantage of the mother's clinic visit to teach her, it is important that the sessions do not cause her to lose her place in line for her prenatal checkup. A clinic patient often has to wait 2 to 3 hours for her visit, and it would be unreasonable to expect her to lose her place to attend class. Arrangements can sometimes be made through the clinic for her to be called in turn from the classroom.

Those in low-income groups or in various ethnic groups may have ideas about father participation in childbirth that are different from the instructor's. Perhaps the father is not the main supporter of the family, or perhaps childbirth is regarded as an aspect of sexuality that is not to be shared with men. Some women feel that the presence of a man would be unseemly and indecent. Lower-income mothers may have more extended family available, and the mother, sister, or aunt might be the one who can give her best support for labor. She should be encouraged to enlist the aid of whatever supportive person *she* deems appropriate.

The educator must be aware of cultural differences. If she is dealing primarily with persons from one cultural group, she should try to learn as much as possible about the culture and beliefs of her students. If their language is different, discussion can flow only in their language. Since an interpreter would be a nearly insurmountable barrier between the instructor and her clients, the instructor must speak the language of her class.

Childbirth educators must be careful not to impose their own ethnocentric bias. For example, the educator may believe that control of one's own behavior is a valid goal for labor. Persons from a Puerto Rican background, however, may think this ridiculous; in Puerto Rico there is a belief that the louder the mother screams in labor, the more beautiful her baby will be. The educators must respect their clients beliefs and work within their systems.

References

1. Anderson C: The lengthening shadow: A case study of out-of-wedlock pregnancy. J Obstet Gynecol Neonatal Nurs 5:19–22, 1976
2. Auerbach A: Parents Learn Through Discussion, p 24. New York, John Wiley & Sons, 1968
3. Packer J, Cooke C: The interdependent team approach in caring for the pregnant adolescent. J Obstet Gynecol Neonatal Nurs 5:18, 1976

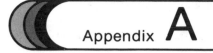

Techniques of Psychoprophylaxis

Physical Fitness

Assessing Exercises

Most women do not get enough well-rounded physical activity to make them physically fit. Although their daily activity may require some hard physical labor, this is apt to be repetitive and require the work of certain muscle groups without exercising others. To attain a healthy level of fitness, a balanced program that will exercise all areas of the body is required. The exercises must be practiced diligently and persistently in order to attain and then maintain an optimum level of fitness. For this reason the instructor must stress the rationale behind the exercises as well as the need for discipline in practice. As with any exercise program, the exercises should be begun slowly and the demands increased gradually.

If the expectant mother is already exercising regularly, she should be encouraged to continue unless she suffers some type of complication such as vaginal bleeding. Exceptions to this general rule are situations involving delicate balance (*e.g.*, a dancer may continue to do everything except leaps when her changing figure shifts her center of gravity) or sudden changes in atmospheric pressure (as in skydiving or scuba diving).

If the mother is not exercising as a part of her customary routine, the childbirth educator suggests an exercise program appropriate for her stage of pregnancy. Changes in body shape, increased relaxation of joints, and strain on ligaments and muscles, especially in the abdominal and lower back area, preclude the beginning of some exercises late in pregnancy. In assessing the exercises to be given, therefore, the educator should avoid those with exaggerated postures or motions, those that force the muscles beyond their natural stretch limits and those that place extra strain on areas already challenged by advancing pregnancy. Breathing is coordinated with the exercises to help keep movements smooth and rhythmic, decreasing the likelihood of jerking or uncontrolled motion.

It stands to reason that any exercise requiring excess abdominal compression is to be avoided.

Another point to be remembered when choosing exercises for pregnant women is the frequency of sciatic nerve irritation. Unlike simple backache, which can usually be traced to fatigue or poor posture, sciatic nerve irritation is a sharp, knifelike sensation that begins in the lumbosacral area and travels down the back of the thigh. It is usually unilateral and is probably caused by the weight of the pelvic contents exerting pressure on the nerve as it comes out of the pelvis through the hip joint. For this reason it is wise to avoid any exercise requiring the expectant mother to swing her let out to the side, especially if the pelvis is not stabilized first.[3]

Physical Fitness Exercises

First or Second Trimester

The following exercises are designed to exercise various parts of the body for general fitness. Individual instructors may have other equally effective exercises that can also be recommended. Ideally, the woman starts doing them before the final weeks of pregnancy. The woman should be instructed to do her exercises at the same time each day, a time when she is not fatigued. Many women choose to do them first thing in the morning. She should dress in nonconstricting clothing and exercise in a well-ventilated place.

1. Arm stretch (Fig. A-1). *Purpose:* To improve and maintain muscle tone in arms, shoulders, intercostal area. *Position:* Stand erect in good alignment (see Posture, Chap. 5), feet about 12 inches apart, chin up and tucked. *Directions:* Raise both arms straight up above the head. Inhale and reach up with the right arm. The stretch should be felt all the way down to the waist. Bounce (extend even further) once to increase stretch. Exhale and relax. Repeat with the left arm. Begin with 5 times, increase to 10 times. Each stretch with the right arm counts as 1.

2. Side stretch (Fig. A-2). *Purpose:* To increase flexibility of intercostals and to improve general muscle tone. *Position:* Stand erect, feet 12 inches apart, arms relaxed at sides. *Directions:* Inhale and extend the right arm above head. Exhale and extend the arm over the head, stretching the waist to the left and sliding the left arm down the leg as far as possible. Bounce once to increase the stretch. Inhale and return to erect posture, this time extending the other arm over the head. Repeat the exercise on the opposite side. Begin with 5 times, increase to 10 times. Each stretch to the right counts as 1.

3. Arm swing (Fig. A-3). *Purpose:* To increase shoulder mobility. *Position:* Stand erect, arms at sides. *Directions:* Inhale and circle right arm around in large circles 5 times clockwise while exhaling slowly.

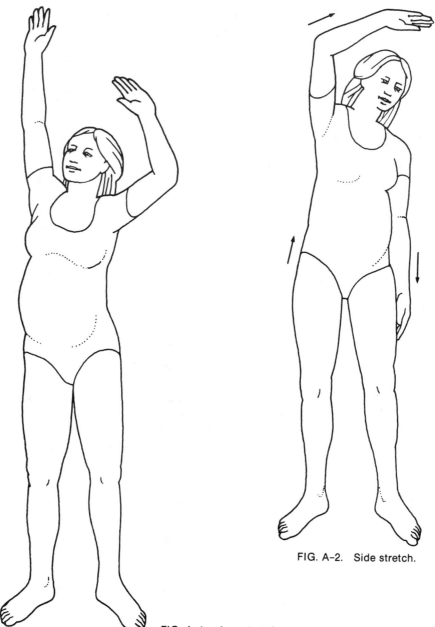

FIG. A-1. Arm stretch.

FIG. A-2. Side stretch.

Inhale and relax. When ready, repeat the exercise with the arm going counterclockwise. Repeat with the other arm. This exercise should be done with each arm going in each direction 5 times, gradually increasing to 10 times. After several days at 10 times, both arms may be exercised simultaneously.

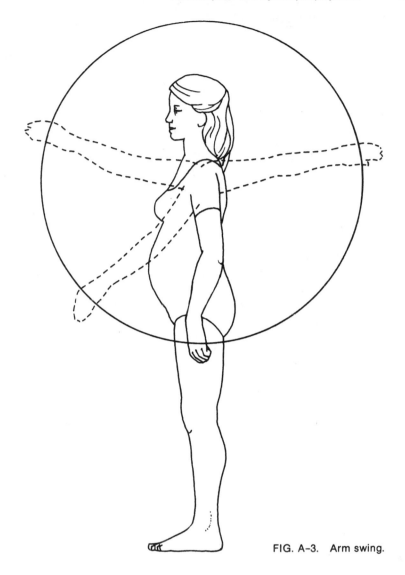

FIG. A-3. Arm swing.

4. **Pelvic tilt** (Fig. A-4). *Purpose:* To strengthen abdominal and lower back muscles, to increase hip mobility, and to demonstrate stability of the pelvis. *Position:* Supine, knees bent, feet flat on exercise surface. *Directions:* Inhale, then exhale through pursed lips while flattening the back firmly against the floor and contracting the abdominal muscles. This exercise should be accomplished without pushing with the feet. Inhale and relax. Repeat. Begin with 5 times, increase to 10 times. This exercise may be improved by gradually decreasing the bend in the knees each day until eventually it is done with the legs straight. There is a slight lifting of the knees when the exercise is done correctly in this position.

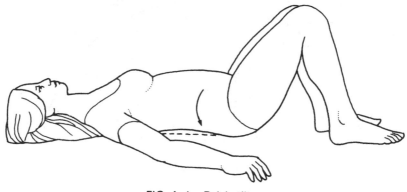

FIG. A-4. Pelvic tilt.

5. **Pelvic tilt, alternate** (Fig. A-5). *Purpose:* To strengthen lower back muscles and increase hip mobility. In labor, to help release lower back tension. *Position:* On all fours, arms and thighs at 90° to body. *Directions:* Inhale, then exhale while arching the back up, tucking in the buttocks and tightening the perineum and abdominal muscles. Hold, then inhale, allowing the pelvis to drop slowly until a neutral position is reached.

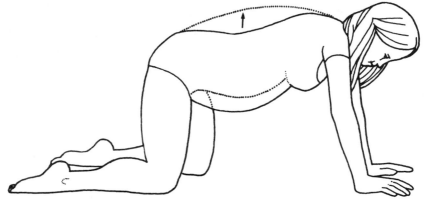

FIG. A-5. Pelvic tilt, alternate.

6. **Bent leg lift** (Fig. A-6). *Purpose:* To improve the tone of the abdominal and anterior thigh muscles and to improve circulation. *Position:* Supine with knees bent, feet flat on the exercise surface, pelvis stabilized. *Directions:* Inhale while raising the right knee toward the right shoulder and straightening the leg upward. Exhale while slowly lowering the straight leg down to the floor and drawing the leg up into the bent leg position. Repeat with the left leg. The stretch on the gastrocnemius may be improved if the mother flexes her ankle while lowering her leg to the floor.

Begin with 5 times, increase to 10 times. Each time the left leg returns to the floor counts as 1. *Precaution:* The instructor should stress the need to stabilize the pelvis at the beginning and keep it stabilized while performing the exercise.

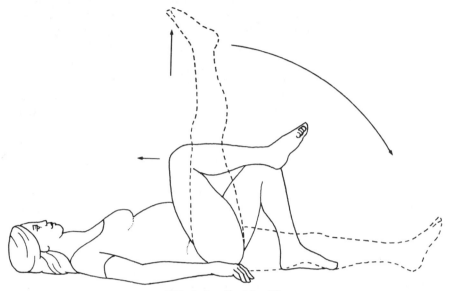

FIG. A-6. Bent leg lift.

7. Head raising (Fig. A-7). *Purpose:* To improve abdominal muscle tone. *Position:* Supine. *Directions:* Inhale, then raise the head to look at the ankles while exhaling slowly. Hold. Inhale and relax. This exercise may be improved, if the mother feels able, by including more of the shoulders in the exercise. In this case the mother slides her hands, which have been resting at her sides, down her thighs. Begin with 5 head raises, increase to 10. *Precaution:* The woman should be cautioned against jerking; she should keep the exercise smooth and controlled. This exercise should not be begun in late pregnancy because it may increase the separation of the rectus abdominus muscles.[3]

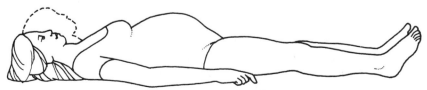

FIG. A-7. Head raising.

8. **Perineal contractions.** *Purpose:* To improve the tone of the perineal muscles, increase flexibility, and develop an awareness of tension and relaxation (important at delivery); to promote postpartum healing and comfort. *Position:* May be done in any position. For teaching purposes the woman may sit on a straight chair with her feet flat on the floor and thighs relaxed. Tailor position on the floor may be substituted. *Directions:* Tightly contract the muscles surrounding the vagina with an internal "pulling up." Release the muscles and notice the relaxation. Again contract tightly, hold, then release. Repeat 10 times several times each day. *Note:* If the woman does not understand how to do this exercise, the educator can instruct her to interrupt the flow of urine several times while she voids until she develops an awareness of what she is doing to stop it. The instructor might also tell the woman to imagine she has a tampon that is coming out; how would she hold it in place? Another possibility is for the woman to practice at home, placing her hand over the vulva to note the contraction of the muscles under her hand. Still another possibility is for her to practice contracting and releasing the muscles during intercourse.

9. **Aerobic Exercise.** *Purpose:* To exercise heart and lungs, and to improve circulation and general fitness. Aerobic exercise such as swimming or cycling are recommended during pregnancy and should be done on a consistent basis beginning in the early months. Because of increased vulnerability in ligaments and joints, jogging is less desirable unless the expectant mother is already jogging regularly.

Third Trimester

If exercises are not begun before late pregnancy, there is inadequate time to introduce exercises requiring progression because of the added stresses in the third trimester and the proximity of the expected date of confinement. However, since the goal is flexibility, comfort, and improvement of muscle tone rather than body building, it is beneficial to teach physical fitness even in the final weeks. The body will be better able to respond to the stresses of labor.

Of special concern in late pregnancy are the lower back and abdominal areas. Exercises should be designed to improve posture and hip flexibility as well as abdominal muscle tone. The perineal area requires attention because it supports the pelvic organs. Suppleness in the perineal area allows the tissue to undergo the stresses of parturition more readily. Awareness of tension in the perineal area increases the woman's ability to release tension during delivery, and postpartum exercising helps muscle tone return more quickly. Also, the adductor muscles of the inner thigh must be supple to remain comfortable in position for delivery.

Helpful exercises from the group described for the first and second trimesters include the arm stretch, pelvic tilt, and bent leg lifts.[5,7] In addition, the instructor may include the following:

10. **Shoulder rotations** (Fig. A-8). *Purpose:* To increase shoulder mobility and relieve pressure on brachial nerve plexus. *Position:* Either standing erect or sitting. *Directions:* Begin by bringing the shoulders up as high as possible, then lower. Inhale on bringing up, exhale while lowering. Repeat several times. Then rotate the shoulders back (elbows face

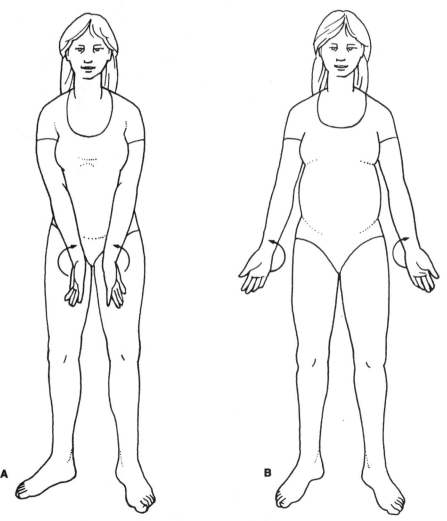

FIG. A-8. Shoulder rotations.

each other in the back), up (as before) to the front (elbows rotate anteriorly), and return to the original position. Breathing should be rhythmic and smooth, in time and with the exercise. Repeat 10 times.

11. **Perineal contractions.** *Purpose:* To improve the tone of the perineal muscles, increase flexibility, and develop awareness of tension and relaxation. *Position:* See No. 8. *Directions:* Perineal contractions should be taught as in No. 8. As an improvement on the exercise the following variation can be added: While slowly inhaling, gradually contract the perineum, rectum, and buttocks. Exhaling again, release buttocks, rectum, perineum, and backs of thighs. Repeat 10 times at least 4 times per day.

12. **Knee press.** (Fig. A-9). *Purpose:* To stretch adductor muscles of the hip; to relieve hip tension and low back distress. *Position:* Sit upright on a firm exercise surface, legs flexed with the soles of the feet together. Bring the feet as close to the body as possible without rolling backward. The hands may be placed on the ankles or under the knees for balance. *Directions:* Inhale, press the knees toward the floor smoothly and exhale to the count of 3. Inhale and relax. Repeat 10 times. The instructor should stress that the muscles of the thighs do the work pushing down; the back

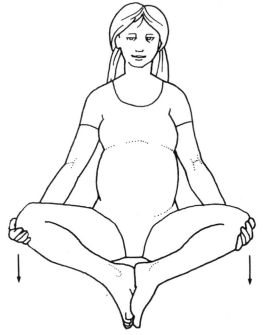

FIG. A-9. Knee press.

remains straight. To improve the exercise for women who are so flexible that their knees press right down to the floor, the hands may be placed under the knees and exert counterpressure during the exercise.

13. **Leg stretch** (Fig. A-10). *Purpose:* To stretch hamstrings and external rotators; to relieve hip tension. *Position:* Sitting upright, legs extended, feet rotated outward, the right wrist clasped behind the back by the left hand to keep the back straight. The ankles are relaxed or flexed. The stretch force is the weight of the trunk moving forward. *Directions:* Inhale; slowly move forward as if a string were pulling the chest forward while exhaling to the count of 3. Inhale, sit upright, and relax. Repeat 10 times.

14. **Aerobics.** As previously noted (see #9). Vigorous walking, 1–2 miles per day in unpolluted air, is desirable. Swimming or cycling is recommended.

Postpartum Physical Conditioning

Teaching postpartum exercises in the prenatal period encourages a quick return to physical conditioning so that the mother comes to expect to do them in the puerperium. It also reinforces the idea of a childbearing

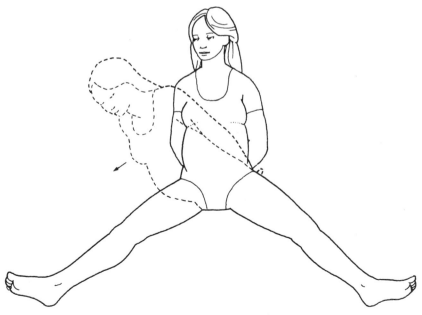

FIG. A-10. Leg stretch.

continuum that includes the whole prenatal, intrapartal, and postpartal period. Beginning gradually, the instructor gives the mother a goal to work toward. Her body will be physically tired in the early postpartal period and it is not necessary for her to make strenuous demands upon it immediately.

The areas of most concern in the immediate postpartum period are the perineal and abdominal areas. Exercises for these areas need to be started as soon as possible. It is suggested that a return to the perineal tightening be begun within the first hour after delivery.

The mother should be instructed to tighten and release the perineal area 5 times each hour for the first few days. This may be combined with abdominal breathing if she desires.

15. **Perineal and abdominal tightening.** *Position:* At first, supine; later, any position. *Directions:* Inhale slowly and deeply, puffing the abdominal muscles up. Then slowly exhale through an open mouth, while contracting the abdominal muscles and perineal muscles. Hold to the count of 3. Relax, then repeat.

Following this first critical exercise, the mother gradually adds exercises that require increasing effort. As in the prenatal physical conditioning exercises, the individual instructor may add exercises that she prefers. The consideration to keep in mind is a *gradually* increasing demand. Individual women may vary in their readiness to increase the exercises.

Abdominal Exercises.

16. **Abdominal isometrics.** *Position:* Supine or standing erect. *Directions:* Inhale, then tighten the abdominal muscles firmly while exhaling slowly and forcefully. Hold the abdominal contraction to the count of 3, then 5. Begin with 3 times, then 5 times, then 10 times per day. This exercise may be combined with pelvic tilting.

17. **Head lift** (Fig. A-7). *Position:* Lie flat, without a pillow. *Directions:* Inhale; then, while exhaling, lift the head until the heels can be seen resting on the bed. Hold to the count of 3, then allow head to fall back and inhale again. This should be repeated 3 times, then 5 times, then 10 times daily for the first 2 weeks.

18. **Head lift, progression.** *Position:* Supine, with arms at sides. *Directions:* Begin in third week or when physician permits. Inhale, then exhale and reach down the sides of the legs with arms, lifting head and shoulders. Inhale and relax. This may be done 5 times, then 10 times daily.

19. Sit-ups. *Position:* Supine, arms stretched up over the head. The knees may be bent if desired. *Directions:* Begin in the sixth week or when the physician permits. Inhale, then exhale, swinging the arms up and over as the legs straighten out for sit-up. Continue the stretch, reaching down toward the feet and bounce once. Roll back while inhaling. Begin 5 times, working up to 10 times daily.

Lower Back Exercises.

20. Pelvic tilt (Fig. A–4). *Position:* Supine, knees bent, feet flat on the exercise surface. *Directions:* Begin after 5 days or when physician permits. (This exercise was begun passively with the abdominal isometrics on the second or third day.) Inhale, then exhale forcefully, flattening the back down against the exercise surface and contracting the abdominal muscles. Hold to the count of 3, then 5. Inhale and release. Begin with 5 times and work up to 10 times daily. *Caution:* Do not use feet to press.

21. Pelvic tilt, progression. *Directions:* After 2 weeks, begin to do pelvic tilt with knees in a less flexed position so that it takes more effort to flatten the back against the floor. By 6 weeks lie flat with the legs straight. When the back is flattened, the knees will rise slightly.

After 6 weeks or when her physician permits, the woman should be encouraged to return to some of the general fitness and toning exercises she began when she was pregnant. These should include exercises for all body areas. The instructor may recommend a book such as *Royal Canadian Air Force Exercise Plan for Physical Fitness: XBX 12 Minute a Day Plan for Women*, published in the United States by Simon & Schuster, Inc, which offers a graduated progression of exercises and is widely available.

Exercises and Techniques in Preparation for Labor and Delivery

Based upon psychoprophylaxis, the exercises here described are those suggested by the Council of Childbirth Education Specialists, Inc.

Controlled Relaxation

Controlled relaxation is the foundation of all the techniques for labor. The skills that the couple learn by practicing controlled relaxation during the pregnancy reduce the woman's fatigue in labor because undue muscular activity is minimized. Since there are no tight muscles to interfere with circulation, oxygenation of the laboring uterus and removal of the waste products of muscle work, notably the lactic acid buildup that causes pain, are more efficient Controlled relaxation can be defined as concentration upon active, consciously directed release of voluntary muscles.

The preparatory exercise taught in class is a valuable first step toward these goals for labor, but it also provides a mode for the woman and her coach to learn to work cooperatively together. The development of a rapport for labor is one of the important functions of the preparatory exercise. The woman must learn how to recognize tension physically and how to release it; her coach must learn how to recognize tension visually and by touch, and how to signal its release. The intuitive childbirth educator can tell a great deal about a couple's working relationship by observing this interchange in class. Does the coach help her to relax, or does he command her to relax? Does he get down on floor level with her and use stroking and verbal cues as learned, or does he tend to stand over her and order her? Are his motions in checking for relaxation timid, gentle, or violent? How can the childbirth teacher help him to fulfill his role as a loving supporter and coach rather than director and overlord?

The teaching goals in controlled relaxation are

1. To develop the woman's sensual awareness of relaxation; to help the coach develop a tactile and visual awareness of tension and relaxation.
2. To use principles of conditioning, concentration, and discipline to teach the woman to release active voluntary muscles under stress (as will be necessary under the stress of labor).
3. To develop teamwork between the woman and her coach.

Preparatory Exercise

First, to place the emphasis upon the feeling of relaxation, the woman is placed in the supine position with her head and shoulders well supported by pillows, another pillow under her knees. The coach should be encouraged to arrange the pillows in such a way that the woman is comfortable, because comfort must precede relaxation (Fig. A–11).

Second, the woman is instructed by the coach to allow her eyes to rest on one spot to enhance concentration, take a deep signal breath, and relax as completely as she can while she slowly exhales. The deep breath preceding the practice sessions will later be replaced by a signal breath with the respiratory techniques.

Thirdly, the coach instructs the woman alternately to tense, then relax, each body area in conjunction with the breathing. For example, he might say, "Inhale as you stretch down your heels, and as you exhale, rela-a-ax." He uses precise verbal cues, either tense–relax, contract–release, or whatever other words they choose, but the cues should remain constant.

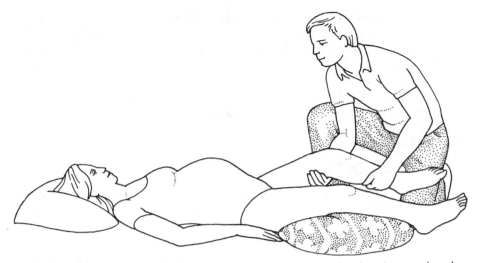

FIG. A-11. The preparatory exercise for controlled relaxation develops teamwork and rapport that will carry over into the couples' labor tasks.

Concurrently he begins the association with tactile cues. When instructing the woman to tense and stretch her heels down, for example, he also taps her heels with his finger tips; his voice is strident. When he wishes to signal relaxation of the area, he strokes her gently and speaks soothingly (*e.g.,* "exhale and rela-a-ax your feet"). The association forms between the word "relax," the action of relaxing, and the tactile cue of stroking. In labor, any or both of these cues can be used.

After each body area has been tensed, then relaxed, the woman is instructed to take a second deep breath and relax completely. She may need to be reminded to focus her eyes on one spot and concentrate on achieving relaxation. The coach now checks for relaxation. The legs are checked by lifting one leg gently under the knee. If the leg is relaxed, the heel remains on the floor, and the coach can feel the full weight of the leg. The coach needs to be careful not to make any sudden moves, because this will cause the woman to become tense. After replacing the leg on the pillow, another stroke assures relaxation.

To check for tension in the arms or shoulders, the hand should be grasped and lifted until the forearm is at right angles to the exercise surface and the elbow is a few inches above it. The coach then gently swings the arm back and forth. If it is relaxed, it swings freely from the shoulder. If tension is present in the upper arm or shoulder, it does not swing freely. The coach must then look for a way to help the woman to release the tension. He might ask her to take another signal breath and consciously relax as she exhales, or he might signal relaxation by stroking the tensed area.

It is important for couples to understand that inability to achieve perfect relaxation does not mean that they cannot use the techniques. It is a goal to be worked toward. If a particular woman has difficulty in learning to relax her shoulders, for instance, she can put more effort into learning controlled relaxation of that area. Because controlled relaxation is introduced early in the class series, the couple has several weeks to become proficient in relaxation techniques and to develop teamwork for labor (Table A-1).

Practice Exercise

Once the feeling and recognition of relaxation is achieved, the next step is to learn to relax all uninvolved muscles when the body is under stress. Because uterine contractions are involuntary, the strong contraction of other, voluntary muscle groups must be substituted for practice. The coach may begin the practice exercise by instructing the woman to tense her left leg (which he taps). The woman responds by flexing her ankle and tensing her entire leg up to the hip. The coach feels the contracted leg to see that it is tense, then the checks the other leg, arms, shoulders, and so forth for relaxation. He also makes sure that she is focusing her gaze on one spot and appears relaxed. He might remind her to relax her key areas, that is, jaw and perineum. When the coach is satisfied that she is as relaxed as she should be, he then strokes the tensed leg and says "relax" at the same time. This practice exercise may be repeated using the arm ("stretch your right hand down and tense your right arm"). The arm is then checked for tension; the other arm, face, shoulder, legs, are checked for relaxation. The right arm is then stroked and the coach gives the verbal cue, "Relax your right arm."

After the couple have become proficient at this practice drill, it can be made more precise by using alternate arms and legs (*e.g.*, "Contract right arm, left leg. Relax right arm, contract left arm."). *The emphasis is always upon the relaxation, not on the tensing or on how quickly the woman can respond* (Table A-2).

Learning controlled relaxation can be further refined if the woman turns over into a lateral position. She should bend both knees, with the upper knee forward and resting on a pillow. This exposes her back so that the couple can work on relaxation of this troublesome area. This position should not be presented when the couple is learning to recognize relaxation or relaxation with one or more body parts tense, but should be introduced after the first two exercises are mastered.

It is not as easy to recognize back tension as it is to recognize tension in arms and legs, because the back cannot be swung or lifted to check. The coach can develop an awareness of the quality of muscle tension in the back by placing his hand on the area between the shoulder blades and over the shoulders, and noticing what it feels like. Then he taps the area while

Table A-1. Preparatory Exercise for Controlled Relaxation

Verbal cue	Action	Coaching role	Rationale
Take a deep breath and relax.	Focus eyes, inhale, exhale, and consciously release all tension.		To begin with complete relaxation
Stretch down both heels.	Extend legs, flex ankles. *The rest of body must stay relaxed.*	Tap heels to signal contraction.	To isolate tension, beginning with a single body area
Relax.	Relax both legs.	Stroke to signal relaxation; look for relaxation.	To associate the word "relax" with stroking to signal release of tension
Tighten your thighs.	Tense both thighs.	Tap thighs to signal tension.	To isolate area to be tensed
Relax.	Relax thighs.	Stroke to signal relaxation.	To associate verbal and tactile cues
Squeeze your buttocks together.	Tense gluteal muscles.	Tap buttocks, or hips if woman is supine.	To isolate area to be tensed
Relax.	Relax buttocks.	Stroke to signal relaxation.	To associate verbal and tactile cues
Stretch your arms down.	Extend arms and hands fully.	Tap hands.	To isolate area to be tensed
Relax.	Relax tension in hands and arms.	Stroke arms.	To associate verbal and tactile cue
Shrug your shoulders.	Tense shoulders.	Tap shoulders.	To isolate area to be tensed
Relax.	Relax shoulders.	Stroke shoulders.	To associate verbal and tactile cues
Make a face.	Tense face; clench jaw.	Tap cheek lightly.	To isolate area to be tensed
Relax.	Relax face.	Stroke face; turn head gently side to side.	To associate verbal and tactile cues; to detect tension in neck
Take a deep breath and relax completely.	Inhale, exhale, completely relax.	Observe for tension; where detected, stroke to signal release.	To make the woman aware of a feeling of complete relaxation; to make the coach aware of the appearance of complete relaxation

giving the verbal cue, "Tense your shoulders." The woman tenses where she feels the tapping, and the coach notices how hard the shoulder area has become. He then strokes the shoulders and instructs her, "Relax your shoulders," noticing the difference in the quality of muscle tone. This procedure is followed with the small of the back, buttocks, and posterior

Table A-2. **Practice Drill for Controlled Relaxation**

Verbal cue	Action	Coaching role	Rationale
Contract your right leg.	Tense right thigh, calf; flex ankle. Focus gaze on one spot to enhance concentration. Think about the feeling of tension in the right leg and of relaxation in the rest of the body.	Tap right leg; feel muscles for quality of muscle tension. Look over rest of body for obvious signs of tension, lift left leg gently under knee to check relaxation; check both arms; turn head gently side to side to check relaxation of neck. Where tension is detected, stroke and give cue, "Relax."	To isolate area to be tensed; to detect tension and signal its release
Relax your right leg.	Relax completely.	Stroke right leg; lift gently under right knee to detect tension.	To detect hidden tension, signal its release, and associate verbal and tactile cues
Contract your left arm.	Make a fist; tense entire arm and lift slightly off the floor. Focus gaze on one spot to enhance concentration. Think about the feeling of tension in the left arm and of relaxation in the rest of the body.	Tap left arm; check for tension. Check rest of body for signs of tension; lift right arm gently by hand, swing freely from shoulder; lift knees slightly; observe face; turn head gently side to side to detect neck tension; stroke to signal its release.	To isolate area to be tensed; to detect tension and signal its release
Relax your left arm.	Relax completely.	Stroke left arm, shoulder. Lift left arm gently by hand; swing from shoulder.	To signal relaxation with tactile and verbal cues; to detect hidden tension
Contact your key areas.	Tense jaw and perineum. Focus gaze on one spot to enhance concentration. Think about tension in jaw and perineum; feel relaxation in rest of body.	Tap jaw lightly; note tension. Check neck, arms, legs for tension; stroke to signal release as necessary.	To isolate area to be tensed; to bring about awareness of impact of key areas on tension in shoulders, neck, legs, *etc.*

continued

Table A-2. **Practice Drill for Controlled Relaxation** *(continued)*

Verbal cue	Action	Coaching role	Rationale
Relax your key areas.	Relax completely.	Stroke jaw and other body areas to enhance and signal relaxation.	With jaw relaxed, whole upper body can relax; with perineum relaxed, whole lower body can relax.*

*Continue practice drill using arms, legs, key areas in random pattern to enhance skills. Always begin and end with preparatory exercise (Table A-1).

thighs. In labor, the skills the couple have acquired in this way will allow the woman to release tension upon gentle stroking of the back. This is especially important when coping with the transition phase or a posterior labor.

Respiratory Techniques

Basic Breathing Techniques

There are two basic breathing techniques to be learned: rhythmic chest breathing and shallow breathing. After the learners become comfortable with these two basic respiratory skills, they will be able to learn the respiratory progression for labor with little difficulty. The labor coach should learn to do the techniques well enough himself to recognize when the woman is breathing correctly and to help her in application.

Rhythmic Chest Breathing (Fig. A-12, *A). Verbal cue:* "Contraction begins." *Action:* Inhale through nose, exhale through mouth (deep signal breath). Use controlled relaxation upon exhalation. Focus eyes on one spot to enhance concentration. *Directions:* Inhale rhythmically through the nose; exhale gently through the mouth to give a precise pattern to the breathing, at a rate of about 7 to 8 breaths per minute. *Verbal cue:* "Contraction ends." Take a deep signal breath to signal end of work period, and relax.

Shallow Chest-Breathing. The shallow chest-breathing pattern (Fig. A-12, *B)* is a learning drill. It will not be applied in labor exactly as learned. The breaths may be described as light, shallow, staccato, high in the chest. They should be done at a comfortable rate but never faster than 1 breath per second.

When the verbal cue "contraction begins" is given, the woman takes her deep signal breath through the nose, exhales through the mouth as she relaxes, then inhales back up to the level where she feels comfortable. This is called the comfort level, that is, where she does not feel the need to inhale or exhale (right where she would be when about to begin speaking). Then she takes small, short, even breaths in and out through a relaxed mouth,

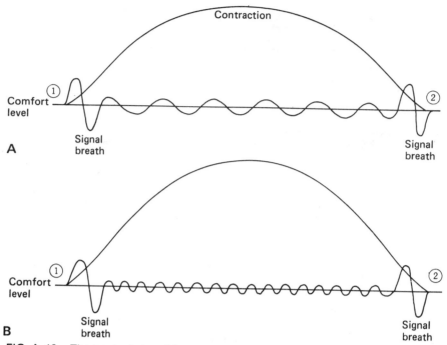

FIG. A–12. The two basic breathing techniques. Verbal cues are "contraction begins" (*1*) and "contraction ends" (*2*). (*A*) Rhythmic chest breathing. (*B*) Shallow chest breathing.

being careful not to stray too far from her level of comfort (*i.e.*, no deep inhalations or long exhalations). For practice purposes she should learn to maintain this shallow breathing for a full minute, ending as usual with another deep breath signifying the end of the work period. *Verbal cue:* "Contraction begins." *Action:* Take a deep signal breath, relax on exhalation, and inhale to comfort level. Focus eyes on one spot. *Directions:* Maintain shallow breaths around the comfort level, inhaling and exhaling evenly at a comfortable rate. *Verbal cue:* "Contraction ends." Take a deep signal breath and relax.

Respiratory Progression for Labor

Once the two basic breathing techniques are mastered, the progression for labor is easily accepted by the learners because it builds upon skills that they already have. The two basic techniques are simply adapted for the increasing demands of labor.

The woman is instructed to begin her first breathing technique (rhythmic chest breathing) when the contraction is strong enough to cause her to tense up either during or in anticipation of it, and controlled relaxation is not enough. She stays with each technique for as long as it helps her. When it no longer helps her cope with the contractions, she increases her level of concentration by moving on to the next breathing technique. Women differ in their application of technique, but as a general rule a parturient should use each for as long as possible because the earlier techniques are the least fatiguing. The puff-blow variation should be reserved for the transition phase (8–10 cm) because it is fatiguing and can lead to hyperventilation.

Rhythmic Chest Breathing.   Rhythmic chest breathing is one of the basic breathing techniques (see Fig. A–13). Add rhythmic stroking of the abdominal area in time with the breathing to increase sensory input and concentration. The motions should be small.

Rhythmic Chest Breathing, Modified Rate.   In modified rhythmic chest breathing, the woman takes three to four breaths in each 15-sec interval, or about 12 to 16 breaths per minute (Fig. A–13). *Description:* Use active inhalation through the nose to the count of one, passive exhalation through the mouth to the count of two or three. Use rhythmic stroking as in regular rhythmic chest breathing. The rate of stroking remains slow. This technique is to be used in labor when rhythmic chest breathing is no longer enough. Contraction begins and ends with a signal breath.

Combined Rhythm.   The combined rhythm breathing pattern is for active labor and should be used when the rhythmic chest breathing at the modified rate is no longer enough at the peak of the contraction. The contraction should begin and end with modified rhythmic chest breathing, but the level of concentration over the peak is increased by switching the breathing pattern to shallow breathing (Fig. A–14). *Description:* The woman begins by taking her deep signal breath and relaxing. She does modified rhythmic chest breathing for about 15 sec (about 3–4 breaths), then switches to shallow breathing until, at about 45 sec, she switches back to rhythmic chest breathing at the modified rate. The coach calls off the

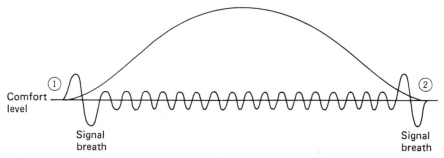

FIG. A–13. Rhythmic chest breathing, modified rate. Verbal cues are "contraction begins" (*1*) and "contraction ends" (*2*).

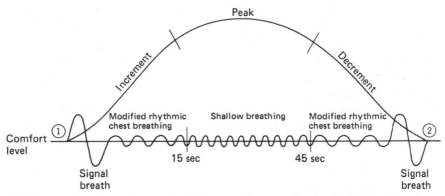

FIG. A–14. Combined rhythm. Verbal cues are "contraction begins" (1) and "contractio ends" (2).

contraction in 15-sec intervals during practice. During labor, the woman will switch when she feels the need. The contraction ends as usual with a signal breath. Stroking remains slow.

Shallow Breathing, Accelerated/Decelerated. Accelerated/decelerated shallow breathing can be considered a reserve technique (Fig. A-15). Most women find that they can manage quite well with the combined technique right up until transition. However, in the case of a prolonged labor, a back labor, or other variation, this technique gives one more option. It is slightly more difficult to maintain than the combined rhythm. *Description:* The contraction begins; the woman takes her deep signal breath and relaxes. She begins doing shallow breathing at about one breath per 2-sec interval. At about 15 sec she increases the rate to about one breath

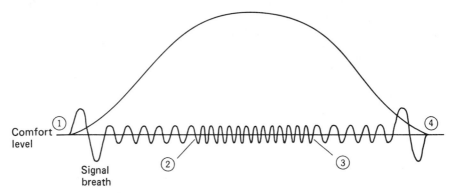

FIG. A–15. Shallow breathing, accelerated/decelerated. The woman begins with shallow breathing at 1 breath per 2-sec interval (1). At 15 sec she increases the rate to 1 per second (2). At 45 sec she decreases her rate (3) until the contraction ends (4). Verbal cues are "contraction begins" (1) and "contraction end" (4).

per second. At 45 sec she decreases her rate again until the contraction ends. The stroking remains slow. A deep signal breath is taken at the end.

Puff-Blow. The puff-blow technique is nothing more than shallow breathing punctuated every few breaths by a short staccato puff, similar to the action used when blowing out a candle flame (Fig. A-16). Because the transition contractions may reach 90 sec, the contraction is divided into shorter, more manageable intervals by having the woman breathe three shallow breaths and a puff. She can manage to the first puff hang on to the next puff, and hang on again until the next puff and so the contraction goes by. The addition of counting introduces a new factor to increase concentration. Most women dislike the stroking in transition, so they may simply place the hands under fundus for support. This technique should be taught in the straight [three-shallow-breaths-and-a-puff] pattern.

Variations of the Puff-Blow Technique. After the woman has mastered the puff-blow technique at the 3:1 rhythm, she may be taught to vary the rhythm as needed when the contraction varies in strength. For example, if the contraction reaches a strong peak, she may shorten the interval and take only two shallow breaths to one puff, or even one shallow breath to one puff. If she feels the urge to bear down (which requires the glottis to close and the diaphragm to lower), she may avoid doing so by blowing out in short, even blows (which keeps the glottis open and causes the diaphragm to rise) until the urge passes. Or she may choose to increase her concentration by breathing in a pattern of 3:1, 2:1, 1:1, 2:1, 3:1, and so forth, puffing out when she feels like pushing (Fig. A-17).

Considerations in Teaching Respiratory Technique

Problems with Rate. The instructor should demonstrate for her class the rate at which a technique should be done. The rhythmic chest breathing

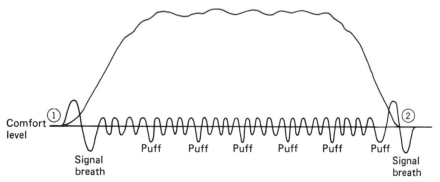

FIG. A-16. Puff-blow rhythm at the 3:1 rate. Contraction begins with a signal breath (*1*) and ends with a signal breath (*2*).

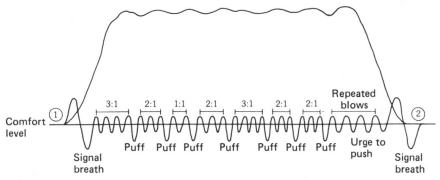

FIG. A-17. Variations of the puff-blow technique. Contraction begins with a signal breath (*1*) and ends with a signal breath (*2*).

should be at about eight breaths per minute, or about two breaths in each 15-sec interval. This ensures that the breaths are neither too deep (in which case the rate drops) nor too shallow (the rate increases).

If the students are told that the correct rate for shallow breathing is 60 breaths per minute, they may exhaust themselves trying to perform the technique at this rate. It is far better for them to concentrate upon technique and let the body set the rate. As long as the rate is shallow and less than 1 breath per second, the woman is not apt to hyperventilate. However she learns the technique in class, the woman will breathe faster in labor because of need.

If inhalations and exhalations are uneven, the problem becomes obvious in early practice sessions. If too much is inhaled, the woman soon feels as if her lungs are about to burst with air. If the exhalations are longer, she runs out of air to exhale and needs to take a deep breath to return to her comfort level. Sometimes she runs out of air to exhale because she misunderstands the need for an even exchange, takes one big inhalation, then simply exhales in short bursts. These difficulties are easily corrected with a little practice.

Occasionally a woman reports actual pain in the diaphragm area. Questioning often reveals that she has read that the diaphragm should not move during shallow breathing so she tenses the area strongly to keep it from moving. An explanation of the reciprocal movement that takes place, especially when the fundus is high, usually calms her fears.

Sometimes a woman cannot execute the breathing as instructed for some reason, such as sinusitis. She should be reminded that the goals of the techniques are to provide a focal point for concentration and an adequate respiratory exchange. These goals will still be met even if she must perform all the techniques through the mouth.

Hyperventilation. Symptoms of hyperventilation may result from breathing at a rapid rate, prolonged exhalations, or repeated blowing such as is sometimes necessary in the transition phase of labor. These errors in technique may be the result of anxiety or pain, or they may be the body's attempt at respiratory compensation when lactic and carbonic acid build up as a result of muscle work. In any case, the partial pressure of CO_2 in the system is decreased as the woman continues to breathe out too much CO_2. Eventually the blood becomes more alkaline, resulting in respiratory alkalosis.

Respiratory alkalosis causes vasoconstriction, which is in turn responsible for dizziness and tingling around the mouth and fingers. If alkalosis is prolonged, it may lead to carpopedal spasm.

The charge has sometimes been made that prepared women hyperventilate more in labor than unprepared women and that this may have an adverse effect upon the fetus. A review of the literature fails to support this claim, however. In all studies, women in labor demonstrated somewhat lowered CO_2 pressure even before hyperventilation began as a normal component in pregnancy. One study found that 75.4% of laboring women had distinct hypocapnea.[6] Since mild alkalosis and hypoxia were shown to be tolerated well by the fetus, it was felt that the "hazard is associated not with conscious mothers . . . but for the unconscious patient who is artifically hyperventilated . . . by the anesthesiologist."[1,2,4,5] It is quite possible that prepared women report more hyperventilation because they recognize the symptoms, whereas the unprepared woman hardly notes mild dizziness or tingling when she is trying to cope with overwhelming fear and pain.

The treatment for hyperventilation is to correct the respiratory technique or enrich the CO_2 content of inhaled air, which may be done by recycling the exhaled air. The woman can breathe into a small paper bag, cup her hands over her nose and mouth, or place her hand about 3 inches in front of her mouth when blowing out. Another way to reduce CO_2 loss is to hold the breath for a few seconds after the contraction is over.

Expulsion Technique

There has been much discussion lately about "exhalation" *versus* "breath hold" pushing technique because of the possibility that the mother may use a Valsalva's maneuver if she holds her breath (see Teaching Considerations). Although we have always maintained that the push starts below the diaphragm, it seems clear that some women do push "in the chest," thus wasting their efforts and failing to exert downward pressure.

The technique and rationale for exhalation pushing is included here. Childbirth instructors who feel that this is an ineffective method for pushing can follow the same steps, substituting the verbal cue "hold the breath and push" for the long steady exhalation.

Preparatory Exercise

As always, the technique should be divided into small segments for ease in learning; new steps are added as previous ones are mastered. For teaching purposes it is suggested that the parturient begin in a straight chair to prevent any embarrassment about the pushing position from interfering with learning. The exercise should be done with an empty bladder. She sits with her thighs relaxed and slightly apart, her feet resting flat on the floor (Fig. A-18). Teaching of the preparatory exercise proceeds as follows:

1. *Recognition of correct direction of push.* Instruct the woman to consciously relax the perineum as she learned in the perineal contraction exercise and to push down slightly until she can feel the slight movement of the vulva against the chair. This should be repeated several times until everyone understands.
2. *Abdominal Muscles.* The lateral abdominals will be used to pull the rib cage downward and to exert downward pressure on the

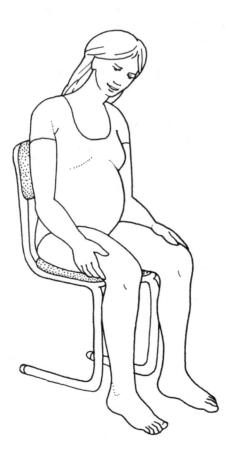

FIG. A-18. Preparatory exercise for expulsion. A hard chair makes it easy to teach vaginal pushing, because the slight movement of the vulva against the chair may be felt if the thighs are relaxed. The chair also makes it simple for the learner to concentrate on each step in the exercise without undue concern about what she may consider an "unladylike" position or about the actual pushing for delivery.

baby. The push may be described as similar to the action used to force out urine (down and forward). This segment should be repeated several times. The direction of the push can be checked by feeling in the groin where the muscle is inserted for the filling in when the push is done correctly (see Teaching Considerations).

3. *Action of the diaphragm.* Instruct the woman to place her hands at the lateral abdominal muscle insertion just under the diaphragm to feel how this fills in when the push is done correctly. Have her repeat the relaxation of the perineum and the "downward and forward" push, and instruct her to add a deep breath, rounding the shoulders and leaning forward slightly. She will note how she is exerting pressure against the fundus.

4. *Putting the first three steps together.* Instruct the woman to take a deep breath and hold it; lean forward and push down with the lateral abdominal muscles; and relax key areas (jaw and perineum) until she feels the movement of the vulva against the chair.

5. *Arm pull.* The arm pull does not serve any useful purpose in pushing the baby out, and may contribute to tension in the upper body. The arms should be held away from the chest to allow for chest expansion. If the woman prefers, she may place her hands on or behind her knees and pull. Care should be taken not to pull the thighs too widely apart to avoid undue stress on the perineum.

6. *Breathing Sequence.* The woman begins by taking two or three good breaths at the beginning of the practice contraction; on the third inhalation she holds her breath while assuming the pushing position and beginning her downward push. She can then be instructed to let the air flow out slowly and steadily while maintaining the abdominal push. When she needs another breath she *holds* the abdominal muscles tight while she leans back and inhales. The sequence is repeated until the end of the contraction."

7. *Verbal Cues.*

Contraction begins
   Breathe in, out
   Breathe in, out
   Breathe in, hold; relax key areas and push
   Let the air flow out (keep pushing)
   Keep those belly muscles tight, breathe in, hold
   Let the air flow out (keep pushing)
Contraction ends; take a signal breath and relax

Practice Exercise for Labor Room Pushing

Now that the technique itself is mastered, the students are ready to move into the position for labor room pushing (Fig. A–19). The woman lies

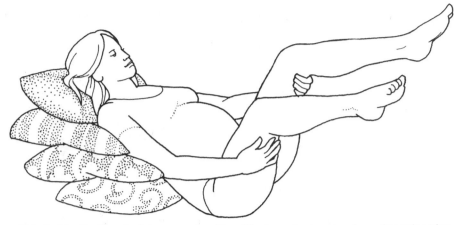

FIG. A-19.   Position for labor room pushing. The important postural considerations for efficient pressure down along the axis of the birth canal are (1) shoulders elevated about 35°–40°, (2) chin forward with jaw relaxed, (3) pelvis stabilized, (4) legs at no more than a 90° angle with the long axis of the body, and (5) elbows up and away from the body.

on a mat or carpet, on her back with shoulders elevated about 35° by pillows. The pelvis is stabilized. Knees are flexed, feet flat on the floor. The verbal cues are

> Contraction begins
> Breathe in, out
> Breathe in, out
> Breathe in, out
> Breathe in, *hold;* relax key area and *push*
> Let breath flow out (keep pushing)

As she begins her pushing effort, she pulls her legs to about a 90°-angle with the long axis of her body. Her elbows are flexed, her chin is relaxed and forward. When she needs another breath, the verbal cue is

> Keep abdominal muscles tight; breathe *in*
> *Hold*

She should hold for about 3 to 4 seconds to begin the push, then allow the air to escape slowly (as in grunting). The verbal cue is

> Let breath flow out (keep pushing)

This will be repeated three times for practice, but as often as she needs a breath until the end of the contraction during actual labor. At the end of the contraction, the verbal cue is

> Contraction ends; take a deep breath and relax

The coach needs to be alert to signs that the abdominal push is not being sustained. He can learn to observe by placing his hand or fingers on the lower abdominal area. The relaxation of the lateral abdominals can be easily felt. A gentle tapping with his finger will remind her to maintain the push while inhaling. During pregnancy, maximum effort should be exerted for a few seconds only because of pressure on hemorrhoids and varicosities. Alternatives include exerting full pressure until the first inhalation, then exerting only minimal pressure for the rest of the practice contraction.

Delivery Room Pushing

The rationale for and application of delivery room pushing are identical to those of labor room pushing, except that the legs will be supported either by stirrups or, where available, by the birthing chair. If a traditional delivery table is to be used, the woman may practice by lying on her back supported by two or three pillows to achieve a 35° angle. Her pelvis is stable and her legs are flexed with her lower legs and feet resting on the seat of a chair. Her buttocks should be as close as possible to the base of the chair. When the coach gives her the verbal cues, the woman responds by proceeding exactly as in the previous practice exercise.

Teaching Considerations

When expulsion is presented to parents, the rationale for position and technique should be explained so that they can understand why correct positioning and technique complements the work of the uterus during expulsion. After describing the angle of the birth canal (Fig. A-20), the instructor can then go on to show why pulling the legs up more than 90° would cause an unfavorable angle for pushing.

Teaching aids might include charts, a picture drawn on the black-board, or even a stovepipe to demonstrate the angle. This leads into a discussion of why the pelvis must remain stable. When the mother's abdomen is neither taut nor compressed, she can contract her abdominal muscles more effectively. If the legs are pulled too high, the outlet will face toward the ceiling and the woman will be forced to push the baby out directly against the force of gravity. In addition, the perineum will be taut, increasing the need for episiotomy. If the mother is positioned correctly, however, she will be able to exert the most pressure along the axis of the birth canal.

The coach is vital at this time. He checks the direction of the push. The back should be rounded, not arched. The belly should move downward, not up. The elbows should be forward and flexed so that the pull is lateral, not upward. The chin should be forward; if it is not, the woman will become extremely red in the face because the great veins of the neck will be constricted, and, since she will be using the neck and not the diaphragm, the push will not be effective. She needs to be reminded when she takes her breaths to keep her abdominal muscles tight. This takes practice, but if she

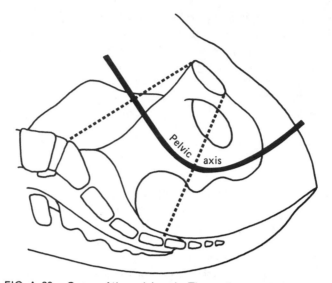

FIG. A–20. Curve of the pelvic axis. The mother exerts pressure by using her diaphragm and lateral abdominal muscles in a downward and forward direction as if she were forcing out urine. If the rectus abdominus is the major abdominal muscle used, as in pushing for a bowel movement, the pressure is exerted back toward the rectum instead of up toward the introitus. (Hellman LM, Pritchard JA: Williams Obstetrics, 14th ed. New York, Appleton-Century-Crofts)

relaxes her abdominal muscles during the contraction, the baby will slip back and need to be pushed down again to the point at which she paused for breath. The coach may need to remind her to take a full breath before she resumes pushing. Above all, he need not be afraid to direct her pushing in labor. His voice may be the only one that gets through to her at that time when she is so involved with her internal sensations.

In order to stop pushing for the birth of the head, she should be reminded to lean back, relax, and breathe through an open mouth or pant.

Of all the facets of expulsion technique, the one that arouses the most controversy is the question of whether to hold or not to hold the breath during pushing. Until recently childbirth teachers and labor room nurses alike taught women to hold their breath during the pushing effort to lower the diaphragm so that it could provide a firm backing for the lateral abdominal muscles. This seems logical because of the increased intra-abdominal pressure resulting when the shoulders are rounded and the diaphragm moves downward. To be sure, some women did misinterpret what they learned and could be observed in labor with red faces, chins flexed against the chest, exerting a great deal of effort in the throat and chest with little effect on the station of the presenting part. Characteristically, when they did take a breath there was an explosive exhalation and relaxation of the abdominal wall with ascent of the fetal head, followed by massive inhalation as the effort resumed.

The correctness of breath holding during pushing was unquestioned until Caldeyro-Barcia began publicizing the adverse effects on mother and fetus.[2] This issue is worthy of exploration by childbirth instructors and labor room nurses, because there are valid alternatives to breath-hold pushing.

When the parturient holds her breath and increases intrathoracic pressure by vigorous pushing effort in the chest, a Valsalva's maneuver occurs. Initially, pressure from the lungs drives the blood into the left side of the heart, momentarily increasing blood pressure. As breath holding continues, blood pressure and stroke volume decrease steadily. Because of the increase in intrathoracic pressure, a closed pressure system is created within the chest that interferes with the return circulation from the legs, perhaps already impeded by the supine position. Less blood is therefore available to the heart.

At the moment of exhalation, blood pressure drops rapidly as the pulmonary vascular bed fills. As the recovery period continues, compensation occurs as the blood pressure becomes elevated to support the increased pulmonary blood flow. Vascular resistance in the periphery is extremely high because a large quantity of blood is necessary to distend the aorta. This means that less blood is available to the uterus and less oxygen available to the fetus. Researchers have linked this combination of events directly to fetal hypoxia and acidosis. [2,8]

In addition to eliminating the adverse effects described above, exhalation pushing becomes a more effective push if done correctly. Athletes have always used a cry or sound to increase the efficiency of abdominal muscle contraction. Consider the cry of the discus thrower, or the "kyi" of the karate fighter. Think of the sound we make automatically when lifting a heavy object. Hoffman's review of the literature confirms the physiological correctness of this.[4] Researchers found that the abdominal/oblique muscles (*i.e.*, the major abdominal muscles used in the expulsive effort) contract vigorously as expiratory effort increases, with the maximum effect at the end of the expiratory effort. Furthermore, the diaphragm contracts to check the movements of the intercostal muscles, thereby increasing the intraabdominal pressure.

A related variable is positioning for the second stage. One of the studies reviewed by Hoffman noted that the adverse hemodynamic effects were markedly influenced by maternal position, with the worst position being the supine. The study also found that when the thighs were strongly flexed, the intercostal muscles did not contract as strongly, leading to weaker, less effective contraction of the abdominal musculature.

Most important to keep in mind when teaching expulsive technique is that the abdominal oblique muscles must not relax when the woman takes a breath. To relax these muscles would be no more logical than to put down a heavy object one is carrying each time one needs a breath. This "holding" of the fetus in the lowered position does not seem to come naturally, but can be learned with repetition. This is particularly important because the woman will be breathing more in rhythm with her bodily requirement (*i.e.*, she will take more frequent breaths during the contraction). The exhalation is a slow, steady outflow of air against a partially closed mouth or throat (blowing through pursed lips or groaning), with maximum effort toward the end of the exhalation. Because it is a controlled exhalation, the inhalation is more likely to be controlled as well. If the inhalation becomes excessive, abdominal pressure will be reduced and the presenting part may ascend.

The childbirth instructor is urged to acquaint herself with current medical literature about breath-hold and exhalation pushing, because new knowledge gives her more information about the safety and efficacy of procedures and techniques.

References

1. Ahokas R, Dilts PV: How maternal hyperventilation affects the fetus and neonate. Contemporary OB/GYN 8:53–57, 1976
2. Caldeyro-Barcia R: The influence of maternal bearing-down efforts in the second stage of labor on fetal well-being. In Simkin P, Reinke C (eds): Kaleidoscope of Childbearing: Preparation, Birth, and Nurturing. Seattle, Pennypress, 1978
3. DeSanto P, Hassid P: Evaluating exercises. Childbirth Educator 2(3): 26–33, 1983
4. Hoffman B: The Valsalva maneuver *vs.* controlled expiration during second stage: A review of the literature. In newsletter of the OB/GYN Section of the American Physical Therapy Association. Boulder, Colorado, Spring 1980
5. Low JA *et al*: Effect of low maternal CO_2 tension on placental gas exchange. Am J Obstet Gynec 106:1032, 1970
6. Lumley J *et al:* Hyperventilation in obstetrics. Am J Obstet Gynecol 103:847, 1969
7. Miller FC et al: Hyperventilation during labor. Am J Obstet Gynecol 120:489, 1974
8. Witzig–Boldt E: Retarded exhaling instead of holding the breath during expulsion. In Psychosomatic Medicine in Obstetrics & Gynecology, 3rd International Congress. London, S Karger AG, 1972

Birth Reports

Abbey's Birth

It was December 8 and our last childbirth class. On the subway home that night we discussed practicing the breathing and pushing techniques daily in preparation for the due date, which was December 26. And there were still many things to do to get the nursery ready—but we had at least two weeks. One couple from the class was already a week past due date. One considers a baby coming late, especially the first one, but rarely considers that the baby will be early.

I awoke around 3:00 A.M., as usual, to go to the bathroom. As I was getting back into bed I could feel a trickle of fluid between my legs. I got up and went to the bathroom again, thinking that there must really be a lot of pressure on the bladder in these last several weeks. As I was getting back into bed the same thing happened again, and as I was walking to the bathroom I suddenly realized that the fluid was leaving the body without any effort on my part. This was not the sudden "gush" of fluid I had imagined when reading about the membranes rupturing, but rather an occasional trickle of fluid. As I sat on the toilet the full impact of what was happening made me start shaking, not in fear but in amazed anticipation. The shaking was heightened by the fact that it was freezing cold in our apartment at 3:00 A.M. on a very cold winter night.

My husband Dick, who had been awakened by all the comings and goings, asked me if I was okay. I told him my membranes must have ruptured, that this was the beginning of labor for real, and to go back to sleep. Sure! I began to get very mild contractions at about 20-minute intervals. Since these were so slight, we both did fall back into a light sleep.

I got up at 7:30 and called my school to tell them I wouldn't be in. Then about 8:30 I called the doctor and described what had happened. He said to come in to the office around 10:30. So, just as I had read in several books and discussed in childbirth class, I decided to have a light breakfast of tea with honey and then take a warm bath while Dick slept. Oh, New York apartments! No hot water. Meanwhile, mild contractions were continuing at erratic half-hour intervals. And fluid continued to leak out in small amounts, as well as a mucousy substance that was occasionally a little pink, which I figured was the cervical plug.

At the doctor's it was confirmed that I was in labor and that I was 4 centimeters dilated. My doctor said to go to a movie and come back at 4:30 unless the contractions suddenly got closer together. That sounded good to me except that the nursery rug was being delivered that day. When I got back home Dick was painting a wall in the nursery and trying to organize in order of importance the things we had planned to do in those last several weeks.

I went to the dime store to buy some slippers for the hospital and some sour-fruit hard candy for later in labor. Came home, packed a bag for the hospital, called my mother, and ate a soft-boiled egg. Small amounts of fluid continued to leak out and the contractions were still mild and erratic. The tightening sensation of the contractions I mainly felt in my lower back.

The security of knowing what was happening made it easy to remain calm during all of the proceedings. It was exciting to think that the baby was really almost here and a relief not to have to worry about gaining weight during the holidays.

The rug was delivered at three, so now we just relaxed and waited. Kissed my husband goodby again, got on the subway, and went to the doctor's. I was still only 4 centimeters dilated, so the doctor explained that the best course of action was to check into the hospital and he would induce more active labor with a drug called Pitocin.

Down to more serious business. We checked into Roosevelt Hospital around 5:30. The labor room was larger than I had expected (we had had an appointment to visit the maternity ward on the upcoming Saturday). A nurse took my temperature and blood pressure, and then did a mini-prep and gave me an enema. It was thought that the enema might induce more active labor, and for a while the contractions were coming at 10 minute intervals, but then they became erratic again.

A little after seven a resident came in to examine me and also start an IV, which the Pitocin would be dripped through. The contractions continued to be mild and mainly in my lower back—back labor was confirmed by the resident, who said that the baby's head was in the posterior position. I was sent down for x-rays to check out the head/pelvis measurements before labor would be induced. Everything was fine and it was exciting when the x-ray technician showed me the x-rays and I could see the baby's head in position and ready to go.

With all the preliminaries over, the doctor arrived at 8:30 and helped the resident set up the Pitocin. About 20 minutes later contractions began to intensify and come at 5-minute intervals. Now Dick began coaching me through the various breathing techniques. It was wonderfully reassuring to have him there, from fetching bedpans to holding my hand during contractions to experiencing the actual birth.

A fetal monitor had been attached to my stomach but did not give accurate readouts when I was lying on my side, which was my most comfortable position. After an hour of active labor I was dilated enough that the doctor could attach a fetal monitor to the baby's head. Now the monitor was recording what was actually going on. It felt good to have visual proof that contractions had peaks and then lessened to an end. During the 2 hours that the first stage of labor lasted I had a strong feeling of security because of the knowledge of what was happening coupled with the presence of my husband and an excellent doctor who is also a warm human being.

And just as I had learned in class, in the middle of a strong contraction I had a sudden, strong urge to push. The doctor examined me and gave the go-ahead to begin pushing. The atmosphere in the room really does change as everyone begins to encourage you to push, especially with my husband holding one leg and the doctor the other. I hadn't practiced pushing enough, and now as I was pushing I would lose some impetus as I stopped for a second breath. I wasn't taking a deep enough second breath so that the second push with each contraction was not very effective. The doctor demonstrated the procedure for pushing, and then he and Dick coached me through the next several pushes. After about a half hour of this we all went to the delivery room and I continued to push. I was so involved in concentrating on pushing that I didn't pay much attention to what was going on—all I really heard was "come on, push with all you've got, one more push and the baby will be out." And I could hear Dick's excitement every time he saw the head. After 20 minutes it really was the last push and I focused on a baby being held by its feet and crying softly. When told it was a girl I was euphoric, although the only outward expression I gave was of my body shaking all over with great relief and release.

As Dick and I watched the nurses cleaning her off, it was amazing to watch her looking all around the room; she was so alert! When she was brought over to us, what was strongest was the feeling of bonding that took place as we three looked at each other. The direct confront of her gaze initiated in me a feeling of motherhood that I could not have imagined before.

Abbey lies sleeping in her bassinet here beside me as I write this. Daily I watch her grow and develop and love her more. All of this began for me with that first incredible eye contact—that is a moment in time I shall never forget.

Alexandra's Birth

April 27 was just the sort of day on which, we had jokingly said, our baby would choose to be born—a rainy, miserable Friday, with end-of-the-week city traffic at a crawl. I wasn't at all concerned, though, as I set off for my doctor's appointment that afternoon. My due date was May 7 and, as there had been no "lightening" or prodromal contractions felt, I suspected the baby would come even later than that.

Emerging from the subway (yes, I was feeling well enough to face the IRT), I ran the two blocks to my doctor's office through the rain, arriving at exactly 2:30 P.M. Just enough time to duck into the restroom, and, as I did, I felt a sudden gush of warm liquid down my thighs, soaking my clothes and running into my shoes. My initial reaction was one of disbelief—this couldn't be happening now, my membranes *couldn't* have ruptured 10 days early! But then, there could not be a better place to begin one's labor than in the obstetrician's office.

My doctor's examination revealed that I was "80% effaced and 2 centimeters dilated." So the baby was definitely on the way. My doctor assured me that everything looked good and that, despite the lack of any contractions so far, I would probably deliver no later than the next day, and possibly even that night. He suggested that I go home, relax, and call him in 3 hours, or, if any contractions should begin, even sooner.

I counted myself lucky that I had rested all morning and eaten an unusually light lunch, also that my bags for the hospital were almost completely packed.

The first contraction began on my way home in the taxi. It was a mild cramping sensation low in my back. With the contraction, the amniotic fluid began to spurt out again, soaking through the pad I had received in the doctor's office and further wetting my already soggy slacks. Thank heavens for the rain that effectively disguised the sorry condition of my clothing as I rushed through the lobby of our apartment building.

I called Peter at work to tell him the news, and then began timing the contractions at 4:00 P.M. They were erratic, coming at intervals of 5 to 8 minutes and lasting 30 seconds or so. They did not cause much discomfort as I finished packing my things for the hospital. Within half an hour, however, the contractions had become much more definite, and I felt more comfortable lying down and doing controlled relaxation.

Peter arrived home and fixed me a pot of tea. We called the doctor at 5:00 to report that contractions were now occuring at a frequency of 5 minutes, and he told us we could leave for the hospital. Things seemed to be progressing faster than we had expected.

By now it was rush-hour and still raining steadily—the worst possible conditions for crossing mid-Manhattan in a taxi. I found it difficult to relax in the moving cab. About three blocks from the hospital, the traffic came to a complete standstill for a few minutes. My impression was that my contractions suddenly started coming every 3 minutes. (My doctor told us later that this was probably due to excitement.) We decided to start the rhythmic chest breathing.

We arrived at the maternity ward of the hospital at around 6:00 P.M. One of the nurses on duty said, "You're doing natural childbirth, right?" and led us down the hall to a labor room. Here I changed into a hospital gown and my woolen socks while Peter went to the admissions office to check me in. (At this point, we would like to say that coming to the hospital fairly early, as we did, has one important benefit. Hospital check-in procedures can take quite a while—in our case it was *1 hour*—and the woman in labor will be without her coach during this time. If she is in a fairly early stage of labor, as I was, it will be easy for her to continue alone with the breathing. In the advanced stages, she needs her husband's support and help much more, and 1 hour without him could be quite difficult.)

Once I had put my "concentration picture" on the wall and arranged myself with all the pillows on the bed, I felt far more relaxed than I had in the taxi. The frequency of contractions returned to one every 4 to 5 minutes. I continued slow rhythmic chest breathing by myself and waited for Peter to return.

A nurse appeared in the labor room and asked about my "pains," then told me a hospital obstetrician would examine me to "see if I was really in labor." This doctor, when he examined me, also asked about my pains. I countered, rather smugly, with, "My contractions are coming every 5 minutes. How far am I dilated?" He said, "four centimeters," and went to call my doctor.

Another nurse came to "prep" me, along with a second nurse who took a blood sample. Both were very cooperative about waiting for me to breathe with the contraction before proceeding with their tasks. There was one surprise now: *no* enema. The nurse said it had not been ordered yet.

Finally, Peter returned and we decided I would be more comfortable in a back labor position. Although I could see my abdomen rising with each contraction, I felt the entire sensation low in my back—almost in my rectum.

The contractions were now occurring at a frequency of 4 minutes, and lasting 45 seconds, although I had some difficulty determining exactly when they ended. Peter suggested that we try the tennis balls against my back, which helped relieve some of the pressure. We were using the modified rhythmic chest breathing.

The nurse returned with a rolling stretcher to take me, she said, for x-rays! Lying flat on my back and trying to figure out why they were x-raying me, I felt, for the first time that day, apprehensive.

The two x-ray technicians were quite patient with me as I struggled to keep my gown wrapped around my bottom and to maintain my breathing. This was difficult, as I had to hold my breath while each x-ray was taken. For one "shot" they asked me to stand and put my hands up on a large gate-like object while they measured my by now undraped back with an ice-cold metal instrument. My situation struck me as amusing—how was I supposed to relax in this ridiculous position? Luckily, they worked quickly and I was back on the stretcher before my next contraction began.

When I returned to the labor room, my doctor was there, and we were glad to see him. He examined me and told me I was 5 centimeters dilated. He suggested that I would be more comfortable if I had the enema, so I did, and it was nowhere near as bad as I had feared it would be. Peter took this opportunity to leave and eat the sandwiches we had prepared for him.

The contractions were now coming with a frequency of 3 minutes, and a duration of 60 seconds. They seemed much harder. We switched to accelerated/decelerated shallow breathing. My trouble in determining the end of each contraction began to bother me. I did not want to pant right through the "rest period" between contractions, but if I stopped too soon, the contraction became uncomfortable. I was also tired of sitting forward, so I rolled onto my side and Peter rubbed my back.

The doctor returned to the room with my x-rays and told us that the baby was in the "breech" position. Between contractions, we looked at the x-rays. There was our baby, with her head tipped chin up and her hands over her head, rather like a cheerleader. My spirits sank. The doctor seemed quite cheerful, saying, "It's not the ideal position, but it will not be any problem, just more work for me." Peter also appeared calm, so I decided it was foolish to worry. We returned to our shallow breathing.

A few contractions later, the pressure in my rectum became very strong and I suddenly felt something *immediately* recognizable as the urge to push. Peter called for my doctor, who examined me and said that I was now 8 centimeters dilated. The contractions were now coming every 2 minutes and, although I still could not feel a definite end to each contraction, lasting about 75 to 80 seconds. We switched to a pattern of panting and blowing.

During each period between the contractions, Peter sponged my face with a wet washcloth and let me suck on the cloth, as I had become very thirsty. In addition, I was somewhat nauseated, so we put a paper bag under my pillows, just in case I vomited. The doctor had turned the lights in the room down so that they wouldn't bother me.

At this stage, which we realized was the transition, I was feeling uncomfortable, although there was nothing that could be described as pain—just tremendous pressure with each contraction. My attempts at relaxation went out the window during the transition, although I did continue to breathe correctly. With each contraction, Peter pressed against my back with one hand and held my hand with the other. (He had nail marks on that hand afterwards—*that's* how relaxed I was!) He encouraged me to concentrate on just the present contraction and reminded me that the transitional stage was the short one.

I panted and blew furiously, certain that my body was going to give in to this overwhelming urge to push. The next examination showed me to be 9 centimeters dilated.

It is difficult to say exactly how long this stage lasted, as I had lost all track of time and Peter was too busy keeping me together to consult his watch or record anything in the Labor Log. We knew, however, that we were close to the delivery, and this definitely helped.

Soon my doctor gave me the welcome news that I could now begin to push with each contraction. We turned the lights back up and my mood immediately brightened. I rolled into the "pushing position" and the three of us, Peter, the doctor, and I, waited for my next contraction—and waited a full 7 minutes! It seemed as though my labor had suddenly halted, just when we had reached the eagerly awaited second stage.

Finally the contractions resumed. My first two tries at pushing were experimental and did not feel too effective. The doctor suggested that I "push from the back" and this helped. My pushing completely eliminated the uncomfortable pressure I had felt. I was still unable to tell when the contraction was ended, so Peter had to stop me from pushing right on through the rest period.

Peter and the doctor each held one of my feet, and Peter supported my shoulders. This left me free to concentrate all my energy on the pushing, as the two of them cheered me on with "PUSH, PUSH, PUSH, Jeannie!" This really was teamwork!

Now the doctor said that one good push would put the baby in a position where he could tell us whether it were a boy or a girl. (So, having a breech delivery would give us an unexpected bonus—a sneak preview of our baby's sex.) With this motivation, I pushed even harder and we made definite progress. The baby was a girl!

During this time there were hospital staff coming into the labor room, but I was too involved in what we were doing to notice who they were or what they were doing. It was time to go to the delivery room.

By now the baby was far enough down in the birth canal that her bottom showed with each contraction, and I was unable to bring my legs together, so it was a bit awkward to maneuver myself onto the wheeled stretcher.

The delivery room looked exactly as I had expected. I was positioned on the delivery table and splashed with antiseptic solution. Peter and my doctor reappeared in blue caps and masks. A nurse rolled up a tray of shiny instruments, and I received a shot of novocaine in the perineum. I never felt the shot or the episiotomy being made.

With the next contraction the sensation changed. While I was still consciously pushing, my body seemed to have a volition beyond my control; it was pushing *hard* by itself. With the last violent contraction, I heard myself growling with effort. The doctor reached in to free the baby's legs. She slid out, and he lifted her up like a trophy as he said, "You have a beautiful baby girl."

She looked, Peter said later, like a silver trout, all wet and shiny. Then she started to cry, and we felt a wonderful mixture of relief, pride and happiness. It was 11:40 P.M., 9 hours and 10 minutes after my labor had begun.

Everything after this went quickly. The placenta, which *does* look like raw liver, pushed out effortlessly. I received a shot of Pitocin and another injection of novocaine for my stitches. The atmosphere in the delivery room was almost festive. The doctor was singing as he sewed me up. Peter and I talked and watched the baby being cleaned, footprinted, and so forth. Then the nurse gave me Alexandra to hold for a moment before she left to go to the nursery. She was, of course, the most wonderful baby we had ever seen.

I did shallow breathing for the internal exam that followed, and it wasn't at all painful.

The doctor congratulated us and shook hands with Peter. I kissed him and thanked him for helping us to share this tremendous experience.

After this, I had "the shakes" for about an hour, although I was not cold or nervous. I *was* so excited that I could not sleep, despite the sleeping pill given me. I stayed awake all night, thinking about the baby and her birth.

Beginning the Kegal (perineal contraction) exercise as soon as I returned to my hospital room really was helpful. I think it prevented a good deal of discomfort in the next few days, and when I left the hospital, walking and sitting were no problem.

In conclusion, we would say that our preparation for childbirth not only spared us fear and pain during my labor and enabled us to see our first child born; it also gave us a truly *positive* feeling for this event. Having the baby in this manner was such a rewarding and happy experience that we felt really good about being parents, right from the start. We think it was the ideal way to begin our family, and we will definitely do it again!

Annotated Bibliography
and Resource Lists

Annotated Bibliography

For Childbirth Educators

Books

Anderson BA, Camacho ME, Stark J: The Childbearing Family. New York, McGraw-Hill, 1974.

Two-volume programmed nursing text. Vol. 1, Pregnancy & Family Health, includes the normal childbearing cycle. Vol. 2, Interruptions in Family Health During Pregnancy, includes high risk and problems during pregnancy. Excellent review for the nurse who is not currently working in obstetrics.

Auerbach A: Parents Learn Through Discussion. New York, John Wiley & Sons, 1968.

Although not specifically about preparation for childbirth, theory and practice of group discussion techniques are presented.

Auerbach A: Preparation for Parenthood Through Group Discussion. Published for Johnson & Johnson (available free).

Excellent handbook for the childbirth educator. Includes discussion techniques and leadership skills, organization of classes.

Bowes W, Brackbill Y, Conway E, Steinschneider A: The effects of obstetrical medication on fetus & infant. Monogr Soc Res Child Dev # 137, 35 (4), 1970.

Concise well-documented booklet including infant outcome with obstetrical and delivery medications, as well as the effects of maternal medications on the newborn.

Chertok L: Motherhood and Personality. New York, Harper & Row, 1973.

Comprehensive study of the psychosomatic aspects of childbearing, including a review of the literature.

Clark A: Leadership Techniques in Expectant Parent Education. New York, Springer-Verlag, 1973.

Group discussion techniques for the childbirth instructor.

Dickason E, Schult M: Maternal and Infant Care. New York: McGraw-Hill, 1975.

Clear, readable maternity nursing text. Excellent review for those not currently working in obstetrics.

Edwards M: Communications: Dimensions in Childbirth Education. Copyright by the author, 1973 (available through ICEA).

Considerations not often found, including transactional analysis applied to childbirth education, ego states and stroking in labor, body image during pregnancy, unattended home births, *etc.*

Haire D: The Cultural Warping of Childbirth. ICEA Special Report, 1972.
  Well-documented study of effects of childbearing practices on the childbirth
  experience in the U.S.
Klaus M, Kennell J: Maternal Infant Bonding. St. Louis, CV Mosby, 1976.
  Intriguing study of the effects of early separation on family development.
  Factual evidence that separation of mother and infant in the first few hours has
  long-lasting effects.
Newton N: Maternal Emotions. New York, Paul B. Hoeber, 1963.
  Monograph about women's feelings toward various aspects of their femininity
  such as menstruation, pregnancy, birth, nursing, childcare.

Journals and Other Publications

American Journal of Maternal Child Nursing, 10 Columbus Circle, New York,
  NY 10019.
Birth and the Family Journal, 110 El Camino Real, Berkeley, CA 94705. Many
  articles of interest to educators and parents.
Childbirth Educator, pub. by American Baby Magazine, 575 Lexington Ave,
  N.Y.C, N.Y.
Journal of Obstetric, Gynecologic and NeonatalNursing (JOGN).
Professional journal of the Nurses' Association of ACOG. Nonmembers of
  NAACOG may subscribe by writing to Harper & Row Publishers, Inc.,
  2350 Virginia Avenue, Hagerstown, MD 21740

For Parents

Pregnancy and Childbirth

Apgar V Beck J: Is My Baby All Right? New York, Pocket Books, 1974.
  A thorough discussion of the causes of birth defects, their prevention, and their
  treatment.
Arms, S: A Season to be Born. New York, Harper & Row, 1973.
  The first pregnancy and birth of a woman who does not attend preparation
  classes beautifully told in pictures.
Bean C: Methods of Childbirth. Garden City, NY, Doubleday & Co, 1972
  Discussion of various types of childbirth preparation and options for birth.
Bing E: Six Practical Lessons for an Easier Childbirth. New York, Bantam, 1967.
  A guide to PPM training *circa* 1967
Bing E, Colman L: Making Love During Pregnancy. New York, Bantam Books,
  1977.
Boston Children's Medical Center: Pregnancy, Birth and the Newborn Baby.
  New York, Delacorte Press, 1971.
  "A Complete Guide for Parents and Parents-to-Be." Good reference book for
  new parents.
Bradley R: Husband-Coached Childbirth. New York, Harper & Row, 1955.
  The Bradley method of childbirth preparation.
Chabon I: Awake and Aware. New York, Dell Press, 1966.
  Good explanation of PPM, including hospital practices and historical overview.
Colman A, Colman L: Pregnancy: The Psychological Experience. New York,
  Seabury, 1971.

The psychological tides of pregnancy on "the pregnant family," especially the expectant father.

Dick-Read G: Childbirth Without Fear. New York, Har/Row Books, 1972
Dick-Read's classic work on natural childbirth.

Ewy D, Ewy R: Preparation for Childbirth. New York, Signet, 1972.
A parents guide to be used with PPM classes.

Flanagan G: The First Nine Months of Life. New York, Simon & Shuster, 1962.
Fetal growth and development in story and photographs.

Guttmacher A: Pregnancy, Birth and Family Planning. New York, Signet, 1973.
Fact-filled book by a leading obstetrician.

Hazell L: Commonsense Childbirth, New York, Tower Publications, 1969.
Family-centered childbirth, including chapters on home birth experience.

Hungerford MJ: Childbirth Education. Springfield, IL, Charles C Thomas, 1972.
Childbirth preparation. Especially good section on nutrition following ideas of Dr. Tom Brewer.

Karmel M: Thank You, Dr. Lamaze. Philadelphia, JB Lippincott, 1959.
A mother describes her experience in PPM in France, and frustration at not being able to find PPM in the U.S. for her second child.

Klaus M, Kennell J: Maternal Infant Bonding. St. Louis, CV Mosby, 1976.
Well-documented work on the studies by Klaus & Kennell of the impact of separation of mother and child in the critical first 12 hours. Includes a chapter on grieving and meeting the needs of premature or sick infant's parents.

Kitzinger S: Experience of Childbirth. Middlesex, England, Pelican Books, 1972.
Psychosexual childbirth preparation with emphasis on psychological aspects. Beautifully written.

Lamaze F: Painless Childbirth. New York, Pocket Books, 1972.
Classic book on PPM by the man responsible for bringing it to the western world. Somewhat dated now, but good historical background for those interested in PPM.

Leboyer F: Birth Without Violence. New York, Alfred Knopf, 1975.
Revolutionary book advocating changes in delivery room practices to allow newborn to accustom himself gently to his new surroundings.

Marzollo J: 9 months 1 Day 1 Year. New York, Harper & Row, 1975.
One of the books written by parents for parents. Wonderful.

Maternity Center Association: Preparation for Childbearing, 4th ed., 1973.
Available from Maternity Center, 48 E 92 St, New York, NY 10028.
Posture, physical fitness, relaxation, and respiratory techniques for pregnancy, labor and delivery, and postpartum recovery.

McLeary E: New Miracles of Childbirth. New York, David McKay, 1974.
Reviews recent advances in reproductive knowledge and management.

Nilsson I-G, Wirsen C: A Child is Born. New York, Dell, 1969 (out of print).
Beautiful pictures of prenatal life from conception to birth. Discussion by an embryologist and obstetrician.

Rozdilsky M, Banet B: What Now? New York, Scribner, 1975.
A handbook by parents for new parents about the postpartum period. Includes discussion of feelings, physical recovery, returning to "normal" sex life, and contraception. Excellent.

Rugh R, Shettles L: From Conception to Birth. New York, Harper & Row, 1971.
Thorough discussion of prenatal development and genetics with many photographs. Includes effects of drugs, disease.

Salk L: Preparing for Parenthood. New York, Bantam, 1974.
   Psychological look at pregnancy, birth, and parenthood.
Wright E: The New Childbirth. New York, Hart, 1966.
   British approach to psychoprophylaxis. Breathing techniques presented slightly
   differently.

Nutrition

Coffin L: The Grandmother Conspiracy Exposed. New York, Bantam, 1974.
   Amusingly written look at how food preferences are formed. Plea for less highly
   refined food in the diet and more natural foods.
Lappe F: Diet for a Small Planet. New York, Ballantine Books, 1971.
   High protein meatless cooking.
Turner M, Turner J: Making Your Own Baby Food. New York, Workman
   Press, 1972.
   Easy guide to feeding infants without commercial babyfoods. Includes a
   section on prenatal nutrition.
Williams P: Nourishing Your Unborn Child. New York, Avon Books, 1975.
   Thorough guide to basic nutrition in pregnancy, conserving nutrients, menus,
   and recipes. Highly recommended.

Breastfeeding

Eiger M, Olds SW: The Complete Book of Breastfeeding. New York, Workman
   Press, 1972 (paperback Bantam edition, 1973).
   Comprehensive guide including physiology, preparation of the breasts, begin-
   ning nursing, problems. Highly recommended for any mother who plans to
   nurse.
Ewy D, Ewy R: Preparation for Breastfeeding. New York, Doubleday, 1975.
   Easy to read guide to breastfeeding. Well written, complete. Highly recom-
   mended.
Gerard A: Please Breastfeed Your Baby. New York, Signet, 1971.
   Straightforward look at breastfeeding including benefits to the mother.
La Leche League International: The Womanly Art of Breastfeeding. Published
   by La Leche League, Franklin, IL, 1963.
   Very supportive complete manual for the nursing mother.
Pryor K: Nursing Your Baby. New York, Har/Row Books, 1973.
   Step-by-step directions, interesting guide to nursing.

Parenting

Akmakjian H: The Natural Way to Raise a Healthy Child. New York, Praeger,
   1975.
   Emphasis on fulfilling psychological needs of infant and child.
Beck J: How To Raise A Brighter Child. New York, Pocket Books, 1975.
   Ways to enhance your child's potential IQ through infant stimulation.
Brazelton TB: Infants and Mothers. New York, Dell Publishers, 1969.
   Developmental differences between individual infants. Reassuring for parents.
   Recommended.

Callahan S: Parenting, The Principles and Politics of Parenthood. Baltimore, Penguin, 1974.
Scholarly review of child-rearing practices.

Caplan F (ed): The First Twelve Months of Life. New York, Grosset & Dunlap, 1971.
Monthly infant development with multiracial photographs. Recommended.

Consumer's Union (ed): Buying for Babies. New York, Warner Books, 1975.
Guide to shopping values for infant purchases.

Dodson F: How to Father. Los Angeles, Nash Publications, 1970.
Fathering as an art throughout childhood and adolescence.

Dodson F: How to Parent. Nash Publications, 1970.
Insightful guide to the parenting art.

Ewy D, Ewy R: *The Cycle of Life,* Vol 1, Guide to a Healthy Pregnancy; Vol 2, Guide to Family Centered Childbirth; Vol 3, Guide to Parenting: You and Your Newborn. New York, EP Dutton, 1981.
Excellent, helpful, assertive approach to the transition to parenthood. Highly recommended.

Fraiberg S: The Magic Years. New York, Scribner, 1959.
Understanding the infant and young child.

Gersh M: How to Raise Children at Home in Your Spare Time. New York, Stein & Day, 1966.
Amusingly written common-sense book about child rearing.

Ginott H: Between Parent and Child. New York, Avon Press, 1965.
Democratic child rearing stressing the art of communicating.

Gordon T: Parent Effectiveness Training. New York, Peter Wyden, 1970.
Raising responsible children through effective parenting techniques and communication.

Harris T: I'm OK, You're OK. New York, Harper & Row, 1967.
Practical guide to effective communication skills through transactional analysis.

Leach P: *Your Baby & Child from Birth to Age Five.* New York, Alfred A Knopf, 1980.
Excellent developmental text including various options for dealing with phases of development, enchantingly illustrated. Highly recommended.

Resource List for Teaching Materials:

Sources	Materials Available
ICEA Bookcenter P.O. Box 20048 Minneapolis, MN 55420	• ICEA booklist (most books in bibliography can be obtained through ICEA) • Film and record directory
Maternity Center Association 48 East 92 Street New York, NY 10028	• Birth Atlas Instructions for knitted uterus
American Baby Magazine 575 Lexington Ave. New York, NY 10022	• Educational program for prenatal and baby care classes

Childbirth Graphics
P.O. Box 17025, Irondequoit Div 3
Rochester, NY 14617

- Slides, posters, teaching aids

Gerber Products Company
Attn: Medical Marketing Services
445 State Street
Fremont, MI 49412

- Expectant parents course outline
- Certificates for class participants

Johnson & Johnson
Consumer & Professional Services
501 George St.
New Brunswick, NJ 08903

- Film: *Newborn*, free to borrow
- Preparation for Parenthood
  Through Group Discussion

Mead Johnson & Co.
Evansville, IN 47721

- Booklets about pregnancy anatomy
  and child care (Especially
  recommended: Series on variations
  and minor departures in newborn
  infants)

Ortho Pharmaceutical Corp
Raritan, NJ 08869

- Ortho REACH teaching aids (atlas
  on pregnancy fetal growth especially
  recommended)

Pampers Professional Services
Procter & Gamble
P.O.Box 171
Cincinnati, OH 45201

- *The First Two Weeks of Life* (film
  available on free-loan basis)
- Other teaching aids

Ross Laboratories
Columbus, OH 43216

- Booklets and teaching aids
  (especially recommended: Clinical
  education aids on mechanism of
  normal labor, obstetrical
  anesthesia, and breast feeding)

Organizations that Offer Teacher Preparation Programs for the Childbirth Educator

American Academy of Husband
Coached Childbirth
P.O. Box 5224
Sherman Oaks, CA 91413

Bradley method

American Society for
Psychoprophylaxis in
Obstetrics, Inc.
1411 K Street NW
Washington, DC 20005

Psychoprophylactic method

Childbirth Without Pain Education
Assoc.
20134 Snowden
Detroit, MI 48235

Psychoprophylactic method

Council of Childbirth Education
Specialists, Inc.
Registrar
168 West 86 Street
New York, NY 10024

Psychoprophylactic method

International Childbirth Education
Association (ICEA)
Director Teacher Services
P.O. Box 5852
Milwaukee, WI 53220

No specific approach
Maintains several teacher training
centers

Maternity Center Association
48 West 92 Street
New York, NY 10028

Psychophysical and discussion
approach

Midwest Parentcraft Center
627 Beaver Rd.
Glenview, IL 60015

Modified Read method

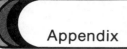

The Pregnant Patient's Bill of Rights and the Pregnant Patient's Responsibilities

The International Childbirth Education Association (ICEA) is an interdisciplinary, volunteer organization representing groups and individuals who share a genuine interest in the goals of family-centered maternity care and education for the childbearing year.

ICEA constantly seeks to expand awareness of the rights and responsibilities of pregnant women and expectant parents. Most pregnant women are not aware of their rights or of the obstetrician's legal obligation to obtain their informed consent to treatment. The American College of Obstetricians and Gynecologists has made a commendable effort to clearly set forth the pregnant patient's right of informed consent in the following excerpts from pages 66 and 67 of its *Standards for Obstetric-Gynecologic Services:*

> It is important to note the distinction between "consent" and "informed consent." Many physicians, because they do not realize there is a difference, believe they are free from liability if the patient consents to treatment. This is not true. The physician may still be liable if the patient's consent was not informed. In addition, the usual consent obtained by a hospital does not in any way release the physician from his legal duty of obtaining an informed consent from his patient.
>
> Most courts consider that the patient is "informed" if the following information is given:
>
> - The processes contemplated by the physician as treatment, including whether the treatment is new or unusual.
> - The risks and hazards of the treatment.
> - The risks and hazards of the treatment.
> - The chances for recovery after treatment.
> - The necessity of the treatment.
> - The feasibility of alternative methods of treatment.
>
> One point on which courts do agree is that explanations must be given in such a way that the patient understands them. A physician cannot claim as a defense that he explained the procedure to the patient when he knew the patient did not understand. The physician has a duty to act with due care under the circumstances; this means he must be sure the patient understands what she is told.
>
> It should be emphasized that the following reasons are not sufficient to justify failure to inform:

1. That the patient may prefer not to be told the unpleasant possibilities regarding the treatment.
2. That full disclosure might suggest infinite dangers to a patient with an active imagination, thereby causing her to refuse treatment.
3. That the patient, on learning the risks involved, might rationally decline treatment. The right to decline is the specific fundamental right protected by the informed consent doctrine."

On the following pages ICEA sets forth **The Pregnant Patient's Bill of Rights** along with **The Pregnant Patient's Responsibilities.**

The Pregnant Patient's Bill of Rights

American parents are becoming increasingly aware that well-intentioned health professionals do not always have scientific data to support common American obstetrical practices and that many of these practices are carried out primarily because they are part of medical and hospital tradition. In the last forty years many artifical practices have been introduced which have changed childbirth from a physiological event to a very complicated medical procedure in which all kinds of drugs are used and procedures carried out, sometimes unnecessarily, and many of them potentially damaging for the baby and even for the mother. A growing body of research makes it alarmingly clear that every aspect of traditional American hospital care during labor and delivery must now be questioned as to its possible effect on the future well-being of both the obstetric patient and her unborn child.

One in every 35 children born in the United States today will eventually be diagnosed as retarded; in 75% of these cases there is no familial or genetic predisposing factor. One in every 10 to 17 children has been found to have some form of brain dysfunction or learning disability requiring special treatment. Such statistics are not confined to the lower socioeconomic group but cut across all segments of American society.

New concerns are being raised by childbearing women because no one knows what degree of oxygen depletion, head compression, or traction by forceps the unborn or newborn infant can tolerate before that child sustains permanent brain damage or dysfunction. The recent findings regarding the cancer-related drug diethystillbestrol have alerted the public to the fact that neither the approval of a drug by the U.S. Food and Drug Administration nor the fact that a drug is prescribed by a physician serves as a guarantee that a drug or medication is safe for the mother or her unborn child. In fact, the American Academy of Pediatrics' Committee on Drugs has recently stated that there is no drug, whether prescription or over-the-counter remedy, which has been proven safe for the unborn child.

The Pregnant Patient has the right to participate in decisions involving her well-being and that of her unborn child, unless there is a clearcut medical emergency that prevents her participation. In addition to the rights set forth in the American Hospital Association's "Patient's Bill of Rights" (which has also been adopted by the New York City Department of Health), the Pregnant Patient, because she represents TWO patients rather than one, should be recognized as having the additional rights listed below:

1. *The Pregnant Patient has the right,* prior to the administration of any drug or procedure, to be informed by the health professional caring for her of any potential direct or indirect effects, risks or hazards to herself or her unborn or newborn infant which may result from the use of a drug or procedure prescribed for or administered to her during pregnancy, labor, birth or lactation.

2. *The Pregnant Patient has the right,* prior to the proposed therapy, to be informed, not only of the benefits, risks and hazards of the proposed therapy but also of known alternative therapy, such as available childbirth education classes, which could help to prepare the Pregnant Patient physically and mentally to cope with the discomfort or stress of pregnancy and the experience of childbirth, thereby reducing or eliminating her need for drugs and obstetric intervention. She should be offered such information early in her pregnancy in order that she may make a reasoned decision.

3. *The Pregnant Patient has the right,* prior to the administration of any drug, to be informed by the health professional who is prescribing or administering the drug to her that any drug which she receives during pregnancy, labor and birth, no matter how or when the drug is taken or administered, may adversely affect her unborn baby, directly or indirectly, and that there is no drug or chemical which has been proven safe for the unborn child.

4. *The Pregnant Patient has the right,* if Cesarean birth is anticipated, to be informed prior to the administration of any drug, and preferably prior to her hospitalization, that minimizing her and, in turn, her baby's intake or nonessential pre-operative medicine will benefit her baby.

5. *The Pregnant Patient has the right,* prior to the administration of a drug or procedure, to be informed of the areas of uncertainty if there is NO properly controlled follow-up research which has established the safety of the drug or procedure with regard to its direct and/or indirect effects on the physiological, mental and neurological development of the child exposed, via the mother, to the drug or procedure during pregnancy, labor, birth or lactation (this would apply to virtually all drugs and the vast majority of obstetric procedures).

6. *The Pregnant Patient has the right,* prior to the administration of any drug, to be informed of the brand name and generic name of the drug in order that she may advise the health professional of any past adverse reaction to the drug.

7. *The Pregnant Patient has the right* to determine for herself, without pressure from her attendant, whether she will accept the risks inherent in the proposed therapy or refuse a drug or procedure.
8. *The Pregnant Patient has the right* to know the name and qualifications of the individual administering a medication or procedure to her during labor or birth.
9. *The Pregnant Patient has the right* to be informed, prior to the administration of any procedure, whether that procedure is being administered to her for her or her baby's benefit (medically indicated) or as an elective procedure (for convenience, teaching purposes or research).
10. *The Pregnant Patient has the right* to be accompanied during the stress of labor and birth by someone she cares for, and to whom she looks for emotional comfort and encouragement.
11. *The Pregnant Patient has the right* after appropriate medical consultation to choose a position for labor and for birth which is least stressful to her baby and to herself.
12. *The Obstetric Patient has the right* to have her baby cared for at her bedside if her baby is normal, and to feed her baby according to her baby's needs rather than according to the hospital regimen.
13. *The Obstetric Patient has the right* to be informed in writing of the name of the person who actually delivered her baby and the professional qualifications of that person. This information should also be on the birth certificate.
14. *The Obstetric Patient has the right* to be informed if there is any known or indicated aspect of her or her baby's care or condition which may cause her or her baby later difficulty or problems.
15. *The Obstetric Patient has the right* to have her and her baby's hospital medical records complete, accurate and legible and to have their records, including Nurses' Notes, retained by the hospital until the child reaches at least the age of majority, or, alternatively, to have the records offered to her before they are destroyed.
16. *The Obstetric Patient*, both during and after her hospital stay, has the right to have access to her complete hospital medical records, including Nurses' Notes, and to receive a copy upon payment of a reasonable fee and without incurring the expense of retaining an attorney.

It is the obstetric patient and her baby, not the health professional, who must sustain any trauma or injury resulting from the use of a drug or obstetric procedure. The observation of the rights listed above will not only permit the obstetric patient to participate in the decisions involving her and her baby's health care, but will help to protect the health professional and the hospital against litigation arising from resentment or misunderstanding on the part of the mother.

Prepared by Doris Haire, Chair.

The Pregnant Patient's Responsibilities

In addition to understanding her rights the Pregnant Patient should also understand that she too has certain responsibilities. The Pregnant Patient's responsibilities include the following:

1. The Pregnant Patient is responsible for learning about the physical and psychological process of labor, birth and postpartum recovery. The better informed expectant parents are, the better they will be able to participate in decisions concerning the planning of their care.
2. The Pregnant Patient is responsible for learning what comprises good prenatal and intranatal care and for making an effort to obtain the best care possible.
3. Expectant parents are responsible for knowing about those hospital policies and regulations which will affect their birth and postpartum experience.
4. The Pregnant Patient is responsible for arranging for a companion or support person (husband, mother, sister, friend, *etc.*) who will share in her plans for birth and who will accompany her during her labor and birth experience.
5. The Pregnant Patient is responsible for making her preferences known clearly to the health professionals involved in her case in a courteous and cooperative manner and for making mutually agreed-upon arrangements regarding maternity care alternatives with her physician and hospital in advance of labor.
6. Expectant parents are responsible for listening to their chosen physician or midwife with an open mind, just as they expect him or her to listen openly to them.
7. Once they have agreed to a course of health care, expectant parents are responsible, to the best of their ability, for seeing that the program is carried out in consultation with others with whom they have made the agreement.
8. The Pregnant Patient is responsible for obtaining information in advance regarding the approximate cost of her obstetric and hospital care.
9. The Pregnant Patient who intends to change her physician or hospital is responsible for notifying all concerned, well in advance of the birth if possible, and for informing both of her reasons for changing.
10. In all their interactions with medical and nursing personnel, the expectant parents should behave towards those caring for them with the same respect and consideration they themselves would like.
11. During the mother's hospital stay the mother is responsible for learning about her and her baby's continuing care after discharge from the hospital.
12. After birth, the parents should put into writing constructive comments and feelings of satisfaction and/or dissatisfaction with the care

(nursing, medical and personal) they received. Good service to families in the future will be facilitated by those parents who take the time and responsibility to write letters expressing their feelings about the maternity care they received.

All the previous statements assume a normal birth and postpartum experience. Expectant parents should realize that, if complications develop in their cases, there will be an increased need to trust the expertise of the physician and hospital staff they have chosen. However, if problems occur, the childbearing woman still retains her responsibility for making informed decisions about her care or treatment and that of her baby. If she is incapable of assuming that responsibility because of her physical condition, her previously authorized companion or support person should assume responsibility for making informed decisions on her behalf.

Prepared by Members of ICEA
Published by International Childbirth Education Association, Inc.
P.O. Box 20048, Minneapolis, Minnesota 55420 U.S.A.
For a complimentary copy send a stamped, self-addressed envelope to
Box 1900, New York, NY 10001

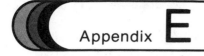

Refresher Classes

If a couple who have previously attended childbirth preparation classes are expecting a subsequent child, it will be important for them to attend some sort of refresher class to motivate and recondition them for this new birth. Unless the time span has been very long or the previous preparation took place with a different partner it is not necessary to repeat the entire series. Elements of the refresher class that will differ from the original PPM class will give recognition to the fact that the couple have a prior birth experience with attendant feelings relating to it, and that this newborn is probably being brought home to a family including an older sibling or siblings. Table E-1 suggests a format for refresher classes.

Table E-1. **Suggested Class Content for Refresher Classes**

First Class	
Topic	*Rationale*

Discuss prior birth experience:
  What went right?
  What went wrong?
  What now seems unclear?
	To elicit feelings; to clarify

Basis of PPM:
  Conditioning
  Concentration
  Discipline
	To remind, reinforce

Techniques:	
Controlled relaxation: preparatory, advanced, side lying	To remind; to review coaching role

Respiratory techniques:
    Two basics; have them demonstrate respiratory
    progression for labor
	To observe techniques and intervene
	  for problems

Questions and demonstration of controlled relaxation, respiratory techniques	Observe, clarify

Expulsion:
  Review rationale for technique
  Observe technique, correct, reinforce
	Appropriate intervention

Movie or slides if available	Motivation, conditioning
Preparing siblings, dealing with two children	Anticipatory guidance

This may be offered in 2 or 3 classes. This general format may easily be expanded to three classes.

Some instructors have resolved the refresher class question by simply including these couples into the technique portion of their regular class series. However much better this may be than nothing at all, it still fails to meet the returning couple's unique needs. A group designed specifically with the returning couple in mind will include both more and less than the regular class in PPM.

The refresher classes should be a minimum of two, preferably three classes in a series. Our goal of increasing mutual bonds with other class members cannot be met effectively in this short span; however, for the multiparous couple we can assume that they have already made the adjustment from couple to family and that they are not now entering a life phase that is entirely new to them.

The initial task is to assess how the couple perceive their previous birth experience. Frequently, empathic questioning will elicit unresolved issues from the prior experience that can be explored and clarified. Feelings about the previous birth must also be ventilated to clear the way for preparation for the coming birth.

If the couple were students of another childbirth educator and you are unsure of exactly what or how they learned the last time, ask them to show you how they remember the technique from before. If they then demonstrate a technique in a way that you find unacceptable for whatever reason, be careful not to denigrate what worked for them. If they have generally positive attitudes, we don't want to disturb them, but to build on them. For example, refresher couples may demonstrate a rapid, shallow panting that does not seem to make sense in terms of what we know about the need for adequate respiratory exchange and fatigue. To comment that this form or rate is wrong would not be constructive and could leave them feeling belittled. Suggestions for slowing the rate or making the exchange more effective might be put into the terms of making the technique easier, or less fatiguing. For example, "I can see that you do that well, and it worked well for you the last time [positive reinforcement]; let me suggest however, that you may find it easier to do if you slow the rate to about one per second or once every two seconds [demonstrate]. Try it and see if it isn't less tiring." Correction has been put into positive terms. The couple can still decide for themselves.

This same general consideration and reinforcement for the couple's prior efforts should be maintained throughout, be it relaxation, respiratory, or expulsion technique. Oftentimes their memory is really not all that clear, and various points need clarification. This is especially true regarding the roles of concentration, conditioning, discipline, the breathing techniques, and positioning and expulsion technique.

Although the couple may know how to do these techniques already, they often don't begin practicing for the upcoming birth until they attend the class. They are commonly so taken up with their lives and with an older child or children that they put off preparation until close to term. One of our important tasks will be to make the need for practice clear to them. They often forget how diligently they practiced to condition themselves for that prior birth experience. If available, slides or a movie of birth can help them to relive the emotions, thus providing motivation to prepare. Ideally this takes place in the first session, but if too much time is needed for ventilation of feelings, fears, and questions from the prior birth, then the film or slides may be shown in a subsequent session. If the childbirth educator does not have access to either of these aids, it is recommended that the couple be sent to a local showing at a hospital or childbirth education group.

In addition to clearing up old questions and motivating the couple to practice, we also want them to begin working on physical fitness, controlled relaxation, and respiratory techniques. In thinking about physical fitness, the mother of a toddler may often say, "Oh, I run all day." This may be true, but the muscles involved in running after a toddler are not necessarily the ones involved in improving circulation, suppleness of joints, or perineal muscle tone. The woman needs to assess where her regular activity needs supplementation for a feeling of increased well-being. A discussion of posture and body mechanics, particularly for lifting and care of a toddler, will also be helpful because it addresses this mother's unique need.

The expectant mother may need a reminder to think about her own nutrition as well as her older child's. Promotion of a high level of wellness will have its effect upon how well her body responds to the stress of labor and how quickly it recovers. A reminder to provide for her own need for rest is also helpful, because too often young busy mothers feel that they "shouldn't" take time for themselves.

In the next session you will want to reinforce these techniques, nutrition, guides, and exercises, and go on to the expulsion techniques. Clarification of the body mechanics involved in moving the baby down around the curve of the birth canal will help her and her coach to remember how to maintain this favorable axis within the birth canal during expulsion.

Another important focus for the refresher class series is the preparation of older children for a new baby in their family. This is a major concern for parents in this group. They sympathize with their older child and want to help him as best they can. What they do and how they do it should depend on the developmental phase the child happens to be in at the time.

It will be helpful if expectant parents think through how they really feel about their older child and their reasons for having this other baby. Children are ignorant, but they are not stupid. They will accept the suggestion that Mommy and Daddy are having this new baby because they love him so much with about the same enthusiasm as the mother would accept another wife for her husband. This is particularly true if the child is still under 3 years of age, because he is not yet ready to give up being the baby himself.

Although the young child has no way of imagining what it will be like to share his parents, frequent exposure to infants can help build a realistic expectation of what the baby will be like. There are also many children's books that will give information about babies. The children who seem to have the smoothest adjustment period are those who feel that the newcomer is "my" baby as well as Mommy and Daddy's baby. The parents will need to help their child to deal with the feelings that are a part of becoming a sibling. The danger is that the child will feel he is a bad person because of jealous or angry feelings. Acceptance of the older child with all of his ambivalence, and a willingness to hear that he doesn't like the baby as long as he doesn't act on those feelings will build self esteem. The more he can use language to express his feelings, the less he will need to act on them. The parent can also help by putting the feelings into words for the young child (e.g., "You really are angry at that baby right now," "You certainly don't like babies today.") It is also a good idea to provide a substitute for the purpose of hitting or kicking, like a punching bag, or one of those blow-up characters with the heavy bottom that keep popping back up. Even a pillow will do.

Special time alone with the older child can be provided by hiring a sitter for the baby occasionally, or alternating which child spends a weekend with grandparents. The older child will feel special if it is emphasized that he can go on errands with Daddy "because you are so big now."

The few days that the new mother must spend in the hospital will seem endless to a toddler. There are some strategies that can help keep time in perspective. If possible, a hospital that allows sibling visitation can be chosen. In this way the child feels included and can have as much contact with his mother as possible. A calendar can be purchased for the child, with the days marked off until "Mommy comes home." The child can then make a bedtime ritual of crossing off the days as they go by. ("After you sleep tonight will be the day Mommy comes home.") Preferably, the child should be cared for in his own home while this major life change is taking place.

Because the young child has such limited language, he has trouble holding on to the security of the concept of the child–parent relationship. A prominently displayed photo of the child with his or her Mommy will help to avoid this problem.

Another difficulty is dealing with the gifts that are brought into the house for the new baby. Unless the child is firm in his idea of "our baby" (as opposed to "Mommy's baby"), this is certain to cause jealousy. Some parents have gotten around this by hiding away small gifts for the older child to be brought out when gifts for the baby arrive. However, this gives the child the idea that every time the baby receives something, he too is entitled to expect something, not to mention the fact that the parents are likely to be found out. They might consider asking friends *not* to bring gifts for the baby in the older child's presence. The most considerate friends may bring a gift for the older child in addition to (or instead of) a baby gift.

Since preschoolers love to cut and paste, the opportunity to use gift wrappings for a collage that parent and child work on together can be made much of, with the baby gift played down. Once parents get into the habit of viewing the problem from their child's perspective, they can be more creative in working out solutions unique to their particular child.

There are many books available for parents to read to the child. A few that deal with feelings are listed in Appendix C.

Glossary

acidosis a disturbance in the acid–base balance of the body in which there is an accumulation of acids or a decrease in bicarbonate

affective pertaining to an emotion or mental state

afterbirth placenta and membranes expelled after childbirth

alkalosis a disturbance in the acid–base balance of the body in which there is an increase in alkalinity due to an excess of alkalies or to withdrawal of acids or chlorides from the blood; may be caused by hyperventilation

alveolar lobules physiological unit of the lung consisting of a respiratory bronchiole and its branches (alveolar ducts, alveolar sacs, and alveoli)

amniocentesis puncturing of the amniotic sac in order to remove amniotic fluid; fluid removed may be studied to determine whether genetic abnormality is present

amnion the inner of the fetal membranes, a thin transparent sac that holds the fetus suspended in amniotic fluid; commonly called the bag of waters or caul

amniotom surgical rupture of the fetal membranes; may be done to expedite labor

analgesia absence of a sense of pain; may be brought about my administration of a medication to relieve pain, which is called an analgesic

anoxia general lack of oxygen, characterized by a subnormal oxygen tension of the blood

Apgar rating system of scoring an infant's physical condition 1 min after birth

areola the dark-pigmented portion of the breast that surrounds the nipple

atony lack of normal muscle tone, as in uterine atony

auscultation process of listening for sounds produced in some of the body cavities, such as listening for fetal heart tones with a fetoscope

biparietal pertaining to the two bones that together form the roof and sides of the skull

Bishop scale scoring method to evaluate the body's readiness for labor or induction; includes states of cervical dilation, effacement, consistency, and position, as well as the station of the presenting part

bradycardia slow heart rate

Definitions for medical terminology based on Thomas CL(ed): Taber's Cyclopedic Medical Dictionary, 13th ed. Philadelphia, FA Davis, 1977

Braxton-Hicks contractions   intermittent uterine contractions increasing in frequency as pregnancy nears completion. Unlike true labor contractions, Braxton-Hicks contractions do not progress in terms of length, strength, or interval

caput succedaneum   swelling produced on the presenting part of the fetal head during labor

cathartic   an active purgative to produce bowel movements

caudal   pertaining to the cauda equina, or terminal portion of the spinal cord

caudal anesthesia   a conduction block anesthesia produced by the injection of a local anesthetic into the peridural space through the sacral hiatus

cervix   the lower part or neck of the uterus, which protrudes into the vagina. It is penetrated by the cervical canal, through which the fetus and menstrual flow escape

chloasma   brownish pigmentation of the face often occurring in pregnancy; commonly called "mask of pregnancy"

chorion somatomammotropin   a hormone, produced by the placenta, with marked lactogenic properties

circumcision   surgical removal of the end of the prepuce of the penis; done for hygienic or religious reasons, or if constriction (phimosis) occurs because of a tight foreskin

coitus   sexual intercourse between male and female in which the semen is introduced into the vagina be insertion of the penis

colostrum   the secretion from the breasts before the onset of true lactation

comfort level   used in teaching respiratory techniques to indicate the level at which one is comfortable, feeling neither the need to exhale nor the need to inhale, as when one is about to begin a sentence

conceptus   the products of conception

conditioned response   a response acquired as a result of training and repetition

conization   excision of a cone of tissue, as of the mucous membrane of the cervix

contraction   a shortening or tightening of a muscle, as in Braxton-Hicks or labor contraction

contracture   permanent contraction of a muscle due to spasm or paralysis, or a condition of fixed resistance to the passive stretch of a muscle such as may result from fibrosis of tissues surrounding a joint

couvade   a custom among some primitive peoples in which the father of the child being born is involved in acting out a labor. He usually remains in bed until the mother has recovered

crowning   time during the second stage of labor when the fetal head (or crown) presents at the vulva

cyanosis   slightly bluish or grayish discoloration of the skin due to abnomal amounts of reduced hemoglobin in the blood; caused by a deficiency of oxygen and excess of carbon dioxide in the blood

D and C   dilatation of the cervix and curettage of the uterus

decrement   the period in the course of a contraction when the force is subsiding

diaphoresis   profuse sweating

diastasis recti   a separation lateralward of the two halves of the rectus abdominis

dilatation   expansion of an organ or vessel or expansion of an orifice, as in cervical dilatation

discomfort signal   thigh or Achilles pinch used in teaching of PPM to prepare the woman to learn relaxation under stress

diuresis   secretion and passage of large amounts of urine

diuretic   an agent that increases the secretion of urine

dyspareunia   painful sexual intercourse

dyspnea   air hunger resulting in labored or difficult breathing

dystocia   difficult labor; may be produced by fetal or maternal factors

edema   a local or generalized condition in which the body tissues contain an excessive amount of tissue fluid; swelling

effacement   the taking up or shortening of the cervix

endometrium   the mucous membrane lining the inner surface of the uterus

endorphins   group of related substances produced by the neurosecretory cells that have opiate-like effects on cerebral and neural functioning

engorgement   distention, as in breast engorgement; vascular congestion

epidural   located over or upon the dura

epidural anesthesia   conduction anesthesia produced by the injection of a local anesthetic agent into the peridural space

episiotomy   incision of the perineum at the end of the second stage of labor to avoid laceration of the perineum and to facilitate delivery

erythema   a form of macula showing diffused redness over the skin; redness

estriol   an estrogenic hormone found in the urine or plasma of the pregnant female. Urine or plasma levels may be measured serially to monitor the efficiency of the fetoplacental unit

estrogen   female sex hormone, produced by the ovary

excitation   condition of being stimulated or excited

express   to squeeze out

extradural anesthesia   anesthesia produced by injection of a local anesthetic agent on the outside of the dura mater; caudal or epidural anesthesia

facilitator   one who assists or makes easier; in group dynamics, the group leader who helps the group to accomplish its tasks

fontanelle   an unossified space or soft spot lying between the cranial bones of the fetal or newborn skull

forceps   pincerlike instruments for holding, seizing, or extracting

fundus   the larger part or body of a hollow organ such as the uterus

gastrocnemius   the most superficial of the calf muscles

genitalia   genitals; the organs of reproduction

gestation   period of intrauterine fetal development from conception to birth; pregnancy

glottis   the sound-producing apparatus at the back of the tongue, consisting of the vocal folds and the intervening space. It is protected by the leaf-shaped epiglottis

grand multipara   a woman who has given birth seven or more times

gravid   pregnant

hematoma a swelling or mass of blood caused by a break in a blood vessel

hemoglobin the iron-containing pigment of the red blood cells, the function of which is to carry oxygen from the lungs to the tissues

homeostasis state of equilibrium of the internal environment

hyperemia increased amount of blood, as in pregnancy; congestion

hypertonic being in a state of greater-than-normal tension or of incomplete relaxation

hyperventilation increased inspiration and expiration of air as a result of increase in rate or depth of respiration or both

hypervolemia increase in the volume of circulating blood

hypocapnea decreased amount of carbon dioxide in the blood

hypotension decrease of blood pressure to below normal

hypotonic pertaining to reduced muscular tone or tension below normal

hypoventilation reduced rate and depth of breathing

hypoxia lack of adequate amount of oxygen in inspired air; reduced oxygen content or tension; anoxia

implantation embedding of the developing blastocyst in the uterine mucosa 6 or 7 days after fertilization

increment an increase, as the increase in tone as a contraction is building in strength

inhibition repression or restraint of a function or action

innervation stimulation of a part through the action of nerves; the distribution and function of the nervous system; nerve supply of a part

intervillous between the tiny branching processes of the surface of the chorion, known as chorionic villi

intrapartal within the antepartal, childbirth, or postpartal periods

introitus the vaginal opening

involution the reduction of size of the uterus following delivery

ischial spines small points on the posterior border of the innominate (hip) bones. These eminences may be felt on vaginal examination, and the distance above or below judged to determine station of the presenting part.

key areas term used in PPM to denote areas of the body that signal relaxation or tension in the rest of the body; the jaw and perineum

lactiferous ducts the ducts of the mammary gland that convey milk

lanugo fine downy hairs that cover the body of the fetus; sometimes present at birth, especially in premature infants

lecithin a fatty substance (one of the phospholipids) found in blood, bile, brain, egg yolk, nerves, and other animal tissues; may be measured in ratio with sphingomyelin to determine fetal lung maturity

leukorrhea white or yellowish mucous discharge from the cervical canal or the vagina

lightening uterine descent into the pelvis

linea nigra dark line sometimes seen in pregnant women, running from above the umbilicus to the pubes

lochia the discharge from the uterus of blood, mucus, and tissue during the puerperal period. During the first few days it is bright red and known as **lochia rubra**. Following this it becomes brownish and is termed **lochia serosa**. Finally, it becomes a yellowish, then white (**lochia alba**) before disappearing

lordosis abnormal anterior convexity of the spine

malposition faulty or abnormal placement or position; in obstetrics, a position not favoring the normal descent of the presenting part

malpresentation abnormal position of the fetus, rendering natural delivery difficult or impossible

meconium first feces of a newborn infant, greenish black to light brown, almost odorless and of a tarry consistency

menarche onset of the menstrual cycle, usually occurring between 11 and 15 years of age

milia tiny pink and white nodules below the epidermis, caused by retention of secretion of sebaceous glands; often present on the nose or chin of the newborn

milk sacs widened parts of the lactiferous ducts found directly behind the nipple wherein the milk pools, to be squeezed, thereby transporting the milk to the nipple; lactiferous sinuses

minute volume amount of air ordinarily breathed per minute

mongolian spots dark blue, irregular macular spots resembling a bruise, usually found over the sacrum of dark-complexioned infants. These spots usually recede spontaneously within the first 4 years

moulding molding of the fetal head by the pressures of the birth passages

multipara a woman who has borne two or more children or who is parturient for the second time

neurohypophysis posterior portion of the pituitary gland

nullipara a woman who has never borne a child

nulliparous never having borne a child

occiput the back part of the skull; used in obstetrics to define the position of the presenting part, as in occiput posterior or left occiput anterior

oscilloscope an instrument for making visible the nature and form of irregularities of an electric current

oxytocin a pituitary hormone that stimulates the uterus to contract; it also stimulates the mammary gland to release milk (let-down reflex)

pain threshold the point at which a stimulus begins to produce a sensation of pain

pain tolerance the point at which the person will no longer tolerate a painful sensation and exhibits an active pain response

palpate to examine by touch or feel

paracervical block regional anesthesia produced by injection of local anesthetic agent into the paracervical area to affect the uterovaginal nerve plexuses, at the base of the broad ligament

parity with respect to the number of children a woman has born, *e.g.*, multiparity, nulliparity, primiparity

partal pertaining to period of time in respect to parturition, *e.g.,* antepartal, postpartal

parturient concerning childbirth; may refer to the woman who is to give birth

parturition act of giving birth

pelvimetry measurement of the pelvic dimensions, done to determine if vaginal delivery is possible; may be done by x-ray or sonography

perinatal occurring in the period immediately preceding, during, or following birth

perineum the structures comprising the pelvic floor; the region between the vulva and the anus, made up of skin, muscle, and fasciae

peristalsis a progressive wavelike movement occurring involuntarily in the hollow tubes of the body, moving the contents of the tube along in one direction

*p***H** the degree of acidity of alkalinity of substance

phospholipid a lipoid substance containing phosphorus, fatty acids, and nitrogen base, such as lecithin

placenta the disk-shaped spongy structure in the uterus through which the fetus derives its nourishment; also, the source of hormones that maintain the pregnancy

placenta previa a placenta that is implanted in the lower uterine segment. Symptoms are painless bleeding in the last trimester or during labor. If demonstrated to cover the cervical os, cesarean delivery is necessary.

postpartum following childbirth

PPM the psychoprophylactic method of preparation for childbirth

prenatal before birth

presentation the manner in which the fetus presents on vaginal or rectal exam; **vertex presentation,** upper back part of head; **breech presentation,** buttocks coming first

presenting part the fetal part that presents first

primary inertia weak or ineffective uterine contractions occurring from the very onset of labor

primipara a woman who has borne one child

progesterone a hormone derived from the corpus luteum, adrenals, or placenta; responsible for uterine endometrial changes preparatory for implantation of the blastocyst, for development of the maternal placenta, and for development of mammary glands

prolactin hormone produced by the anterior pituitary gland, capable of initiating and sustaining lactation when other essential hormones such as estrogen, progesterone, and oxytocin are present

prolapse a falling or dropping down of an organ such as the uterus

prostaglandin an extremely active biological substance normally present in many body tissues, which causes smooth muscle to contract; currently being studied for use in induction of labor and for abortion

psychoprophylaxis physical and psychological preparation for childbirth; PPM

pudendal block regional anesthesia produced by injecting a local anesthetic agent into the pudendal nerve plexus either transvaginally or through the buttock

puerperium   the period of 42 days following childbirth; the generative organs usually return to normal within this time

quickening   first movements of the fetus felt *in utero*

respiratory distress syndrome (RDS)   hyaline membrane disease. Clinical signs include delayed onset of respiration and low Apgar score. Etiology is unknown, but prematurity is a predisposing factor.

rugae   a fold or crease, especially in mucous membrane, such as on the inner surface of the vagina

saddle block   a low spinal block to anesthetize the perineum and buttocks area

sciatic nerve   largest nerve in the body, arising from the sacral plexus, leaving the pelvis through the greater sciatic foramen, running through the hip joint and down the back of the thigh. Sciatic nerve irritation is common during pregnancy.

secondary inertia   weak or ineffective uterine contractions following prolonged labor, with maternal exhaustion

semen   a thick, viscid secretion discharged from the urethra of the male at orgasm, containing the spermatozoa

signal breath   term used in PPM to denote the beginning or end of the work period (or contraction)

sitz bath   bath to sit in with water covering the hips

sonography (ultrasonography)   use of ultrasound to produce an image or photograph of an organ or tissue; ultrasonic echoes are recorded as they strike tissues of varying densities

sphingomyelin   a phosphorous-containing lipid; the ratio of lecithin to sphingomyelin may be measured by obtaining fluid through amniocentesis to assess the maturity of the fetal lungs

spinal   pertaining to the spine or spinal cord

spinal anesthesia   anesthesia produced by injection of anesthetic into the spinal canal

stasis   stagnation of the normal flow of fluids

station   measurement of descent of the presenting part in relation to the ischial spines

striae gravidarum   stretch marks; fine pinkish lines seen over the abdomen and sometimes the breasts of pregnant women. These recede following delivery and become silvery white

subinvolution   incomplete return of a part to normal dimensions, such as the uterus following childbirth

substantia gelatinosa   gray matter of the cord surrounding the central canal and capping the head of the posterior horns of the spinal cord

surfactant   an agent that lowers surface tension. Pulmonary surfactant is produced beginning at 35–36 weeks' gestation by the fetal alveolar cells. Its role is to maintain the stability of the alveolus so that it does not collapse on expiration

symphysis pubis   the junction of the pubic bones on midline in front

synapse   the point of junction of two neurons in a neural pathway; synapses are the contact point where an impulse traveling in one neuron initiates an impulse in the second. The synaptic ability may be altered by fatigue, chemical changes such as with anesthetics, or oxygen deficiency.

tachycardia   abnormally rapid heart rate

tailor sitting   sitting with both knees flexed and ankles crossed

teratogen   anything that causes the development of abnormal structures in the embryo or fetus, *e.g.,* thalidomide

thalamus   the largest subdivision of the diencephalon, whose function is to receive all sensory stimuli with the exception of olfactory. The thalamus is also the center for appreciation of primitive uncritical sensations of pain, crude touch, and temperature, before the impulse has reached the cerebral cortex for interpretation

tonus   the quality of muscle tension that determines firmness or flaccidity

transducer   a device that converts one form of energy to another; used in ultrasonography to receive the energy produced by sound waves and relay it to another transducer that makes a record of it on a recording device

ultrasound   ultrasound waves have different velocities in tissues that differ in density and elasticity from others. This property permits outlining the shape of various tissues within the body, such as the fetal parts, fetal size and position, *etc.*

umbilicus   a scar in the center of the abdomen that marks the point where the umbilical cord was attached *in utero*

varicosity   a swollen, twisted vein

vasoconstriction   constriction of the blood vessels

vernix caseosa   a hand-cream-like sebaceous substance that protected the fetal skin *in utero* and may be seen at birth; most abundant in creases, it is unnecessary to remove it

viscera   internal organs

Index

The letter *f* following a page number represents a figure; *t* indicates tabular material. Numbers in **boldface** indicate glossary definitions.